More Praise for *SIT UP STRAIGHT*

"My body was wrecked after four seasons of shooting *Into the Badlands*. . . . In just four sessions Vinh 'fixed' me! Besides the amazing treatment, what I appreciated is that he gave me exercises I could take home to, literally, get me straight. You may not be a martial artist or even a high-level athlete, but I can guarantee that you're doing something in your daily routine that isn't good for your body. . . . *Sit Up Straight* teaches you how to 'futureproof.'"

—Daniel Wu, executive producer and star of AMC's *Into the Badlands*

"The kind of twisting that athletes must do to win snowboarding medals isn't possible without maximum flexibility. Your movement goals may not involve competing at the X Games, but if you want to understand how your body works and how you can make it work for you in the future, read Vinh's book."

—Chloe Kim, World, Olympic, and X Games halfpipe champion

"Vinh Pham is one of those with 'the knowledge.' Listen to him. He'll save you from pain, and help you push past what you thought were your limits."

**—Joe De Sena, *New York Times* bestselling author of *Spartan UP!*
and executive producer of NBC's *Spartan: Ultimate Team Challenge***

"A wonderful book . . . As a trainer, I'm all about having fun. But you can't have fun if you're in pain. *Sit Up Straight* is a mobility map that steers us away from pain and closer to our best self. Read it! Your body will thank you!"

**—Kaisa Keranen, founder of Just Move, frequently seen
in such magazines as *Vogue*, *Shape*, and *Self***

"This book can dramatically affect the person you'll be years from now. Vinh delivers quick and effective movements that won't take much time and can easily be implemented."

**—Jen Esquer, DPT, ranked one of the best physical therapy trainers
on Instagram by *Shape* magazine *and* cohost of *The Optimal Body* podcast**

"*Sit Up Straight* offers a lot more than the admonition in the title. (Spoiler alert: Your mom wasn't wrong.) Its posture-improving exercises show you where you lack mobility and stability, giving you valuable tools to fix the problems you have and prevent the ones you're at risk of developing."

**—Lou Schuler, National Magazine Award–winning journalist,
former fitness director at *Men's Health*, and author of *The New Rules of Lifting***

"Performing at a high level in the gym—or just getting through life without pain—is about more than willing yourself to finish. It's about understanding how body part A works with body part B. No one knows that better than Vinh. His book is a road map to a life of no limitations."

—Ron Boss Everline, entrepreneur and fitness trainer

"This book asks you to get honest with yourself about the daily toll you're taking on your body. . . . *Sit Up Straight* isn't just for the slouchers among us. It's an insight-filled manual for anyone with muscles and joints—yes, that's *all* of us—who wants to remain pain-free. Integrating this daily into your life can make a big difference!"

—Chris Mohr, PhD, RD, co-owner of well-being
consulting company Mohr Results, Inc.

"Keeping your body in good alignment and health not only allows you to move freely but helps all the intricate systems in your body work in harmony. Vinh is a movement expert who'll teach you new things. . . . Read his book now and you'll be reaping the rewards *years* from now."

—Fai Khadra, artist

SIT UP STRAIGHT

Futureproof Your Body Against Chronic Pain with 12 Simple Movements

VINH PHAM

with
Jeff O'Connell

SCRIBNER

New York London Toronto Sydney New Delhi

Scribner
An Imprint of Simon & Schuster, Inc.
1230 Avenue of the Americas
New York, NY 10020

First Scribner hardcover edition April 2022

SCRIBNER and design are registered trademarks of The Gale Group, Inc., used under license by Simon & Schuster, Inc., the publisher of this work.

For information about special discounts for bulk purchases, please contact Simon & Schuster Special Sales at 1-866-506-1949 or business@simonandschuster.com.

The Simon & Schuster Speakers Bureau can bring authors to your live event. For more information or to book an event, contact the Simon & Schuster Speakers Bureau at 1-866-248-3049 or visit our website at www.simonspeakers.com.

Interior design by Jason Snyder

Manufactured in the United States of America

3 5 7 9 10 8 6 4 2

Library of Congress Cataloging-in-Publication Data has been applied for.

ISBN 978-1-9821-8156-7
ISBN 978-1-9821-8158-1 (ebook)

For the Myodetox tribe

CONTENTS

PREFACE

IN EARLY 2020, before the coronavirus shut down the world, I raised money to expand the North American footprint of Myodetox. As part of that process, I spent a lot of time meeting with investors and dealmakers. This was high-level networking of the sort that suits my outgoing personality. I love meeting people and exchanging ideas and opportunities. I feed off that energy and creativity. It makes me feel as if I've plugged into some mysterious energy source.

Though I've been a physical therapist since 2007, I never thought my work would lead to me being introduced to a powerful tech-industry lawyer—someone used to executing mergers and acquisitions involving billions of dollars. This lawyer was a promising enough connection that, after he and I spoke by phone, my Myodetox team and I flew to San Francisco for the sole purpose of meeting with him. As part of the visit, we scheduled a Myodetox session to take place in his office, the goal being to further his understanding of exactly what it is I do.

After arriving at the airport, my colleagues and I made our way to his office, located in a futuristic-looking high-rise soaring above the downtown financial district. The elevator swooshed up to the fiftieth floor and stopped with a beep; as we stepped out, smiling staffers whisked us inside.

After choosing from among what seemed like several dozen flavors of coffee, I was led into the lawyer's corner office, which offered a sweeping view of downtown San Francisco. It's the sort of view that I'm sure makes the occupant feel like a master of the universe. The lawyer came out from behind his desk to greet me. The office walls were practically papered with degrees; in various corners, piles of documents were stacked high.

First, we talked about business. He wanted to know more about what Myodetox does and what—beyond our more contemporary vibe—differentiates us from our competitors. I explained that we're a chain of physical therapy clinics with an innovative approach to treating patients: Rather than waiting for patients to come to us in pain, our team works to prevent injury altogether by futureproofing the body. Our mission is to make healthcare accessible to everyone by making "self-care" a lifestyle.

Eventually the conversation turned to the lawyer's own body. Suddenly he transformed from a brilliant, self-assured tech titan to a person speaking about his body with about as much understanding as a five-year-old playing Operation. "My back has really been bothering me lately," he said. "It's this part right here. Do you know what that is?"

It was the lumbar spine, a pretty basic part of the human anatomy.

"Can you sit up straight?" I asked. When patients come to me with back issues, this is always one of the first things I ask. How your spine looks when sitting tall is often a tell to what's causing the pain.

After I spent a few minutes talking with the lawyer about the importance of maintaining a strong posture—especially crucial for someone like him, who sat for most of the day—as well as other techniques like engaging the core muscles and doing some light treatment, I blurted out something that was probably less than diplomatic.

"You're one of the smartest people I've ever met," I said, "yet you have to ask a random bearded Asian guy from Toronto how your back works?"

I explained that I wasn't trying to make him feel bad, but that the issue he was facing was exactly what I was trying to solve with my company: how to increase the baseline knowledge people have of their own bodies. I firmly believe that people should have at least a rudimentary understanding of the only thing they truly own.

I want to get them out of pain, futureproofing their bodies so they can maximize their full potential and live longer.

Part of building a business like mine is meeting with numerous investors and VIPs. Most are type A, and many are brilliant. I've noticed a commonality, though, in meeting with them individually, as I did with that tech-industry lawyer. Many have made enormous sacrifices to fulfill their business dreams, but what they've sacrificed above all else is their health. They worked hard, relentlessly attending to every business detail, yet paid little heed to their own body. Until one day, surrounded by success and wealth, they woke up and realized that their body had betrayed them. Or, rather, they'd betrayed their body. Because they ignored it.

The sad result is that they don't even have the opportunity to enjoy the fruits of their labor. They're saddled with health issues and chronic pain, spending much of their free time (and hard-earned money) in the doctor's office rather than on the links or playing with their grandkids. It's the biggest regret most of these high achievers have.

I'll be the first to admit that I've been guilty of this, too. I ignored my body in my early years to build my company. To stop this downward spiral, I had to create a better way to take care of my body—it's called futureproofing. The key is following a posture hygiene plan that isn't much more complicated than brushing and flossing your teeth every day. Think of it as "brushing your spine" and "flossing your muscles." It's not hard, but you have to do it every day to avoid problems down the road.

See, the most valuable possession you own is your body. The more time you spend taking care of your health regularly earlier, the less time you'll spend being sick and unable to move later. Conversely, the less time you spend taking care of your health, the more time you'll eventually spend ill and partially or completely immobile.

The idea that a person must choose between the two—either health or success—was always a false choice, anyway. Taking better care of your body can make you even *more* successful in life.

So it's time to take charge and take care of your body like a boss—a benevolent and inspiring leader, not the one you tune out because they're discouraging. Have you ever felt ignored at work? Imagine how your knee feels. When was the last time you checked in with your muscles and joints? I'm guessing you make regular trips to the doctor and dentist for checkups and preventive care (or at least I hope you do). Usually, the nurse measures your blood pressure and the dental assistant takes X-rays even in the absence of symptoms; monitoring your internal systems for trouble is simply a default. But when was the last time you visited someone to see if your knee was working well? Do you even *know* which muscles control your knee? Do you pay attention to any of the muscles that work tirelessly for you every day from morning to night, taking you where you need to go?

Before you beat yourself up too badly, I'll point out that you have a partial excuse. There's so much material out there about losing weight, building muscle, and gaining strength, but so little on injury prevention and movement optimization. Even the books that are written on the subject are geared toward experts (personal trainers or physical therapists). There's precious little information available for the average person. So this book collects everything I've learned from taking classes, treating patients, and talking with other experts in the field—and I convey it with a simplicity that eliminates the need to obtain an advanced degree in physiology.

It's important to keep this in mind: If you break, you can't help others. My parents' generation was always about taking care of other people. Now the new buzzword is *self-care*. At first, you might think self-care is selfish and self-absorbed, the glorification of oneself. But self-care is actually about making sure you're healthy so you can be *more* effective at taking care of others, just as you're supposed to put on your own oxygen mask before helping others on a plane.

Time may never be your ally, but it doesn't have to be your enemy. Follow this plan, and you and time can achieve a truce, one that allows you to pursue your dreams, enjoy good health, and make your mark on the world.

1 POSTURE, PAIN, AND A PANDEMIC

GIVEN THAT YOU OPENED or downloaded this book, I'm guessing your days of feeling 100 percent have been growing increasingly rare. Maybe your neck feels achy and stiff, to the point that the simple act of turning your head from side to side makes a sound like milk hitting a bowl of Rice Krispies. Perhaps your back aches down around the tailbone and higher up as well. After you've been staring at a screen for any length of time, a dull ache forms, so you massage your temples for relief. Eventually that dull ache becomes a steady drumbeat that makes you reach for a bottle of aspirin or something more powerful.

Why does it have to be this way? When did life stop being fun and effortless? What the hell is wrong with me?

When you stand up and begin moving around, your hips resist. This tightness has changed the way you walk, although it's happened so gradually that you don't even realize it—until you catch a glimpse of yourself in a window's reflection, and your gait doesn't look free and effortless like it once did. The swagger of youth has given way to the creakiness of old age, which may seem inevitable, except . . . you're not old yet. You only *look* and *feel* old. You're starting to move the stiff way your parents did. You try to reach down and touch your toes, but, *argh*, jolts of pain shoot up the back of your hamstrings. Stretch the muscles on the back of your leg any farther and they threaten to snap like rubber bands pulled past their limit.

That's just the start of the issues plaguing you around the clock, though. You wonder, *Where did my energy go?* You used to work so much and play so hard that you forgot to sleep half the time. Now nine o'clock isn't the start of your evening; it's bedtime. It feels like someone unplugged your body from a wall socket. You're so irritable that your friends and family feel like they're walking on eggshells around you. Your digestion feels sluggish and incomplete; it's as though there's a traffic jam in your colon and your stomach is bickering with your brain.

All these issues and more have begun playing with your mind in ways that have you questioning your self-worth. It's hard to decipher what's causing what. You know exercise is one way to regain control of your life and body, yet all your symptoms make working out seem like a Herculean task. *This hole I'm in feels so deep,* you keep thinking, yearning for the days when your body worked instinctively. Now you view everything through the prism of your pain, discomfort, and lack of mobility, and it sucks.

One question lingers: *Can I get back to where I was? Or is it all downhill from here?*

I'm here to answer yes to the first question, and no to the second. I've seen it myself with literally hundreds of patients I've treated over the years.

One of those patients illustrates what I mean. On a fall morning in 2010, a nurse named Nancy Elliott came to see me in Toronto for physical therapy. She was hunched over and shuffled her feet, moving as though she were eighty years old, not fifty, as her chart indicated. A short way into my exam, I learned that she'd been dealing with crippling bursitis in her hips for years and that I was the fourteenth medical doctor or physical therapist she'd seen.

Despite all of this previous medical attention, Nancy had actually gotten worse, not better, under care. Her hips ached on both sides, preventing her from sleeping for more than brief interludes. And to make matters worse, the painkillers, cortisone shots, and other drugs she'd taken had left her with terrible stomach issues. She felt awful. Doctors had suggested operating in an attempt to reduce her pain, but she clung to the hope that it was possible to feel better without resorting to surgery.

I wanted to see how she walked. As Nancy rose gingerly from the examination table and began moving across the room, her feet splayed outward like a duck. This simple task seemed to overwhelm her. Finally she maneuvered herself back to a chair, wincing as she sat back down.

"Oh my God, I'm miserable," Nancy admitted.

Later she told me I was the first practitioner who'd bothered asking to see how she walked. "None of them asked—not the orthopedic doctor, not even the physiotherapist I saw three times a week for over a year. They all asked, 'Where are you sore?' before focusing on that area. But it wasn't helpful. It didn't reduce my pain."

I was interested in her gait and her posture, and what I observed was a prescription for the issues she was experiencing. Both Nancy's posture and movement were a mess because she'd developed several bad habits to compensate for her original set of problems, one habit compounding the next.

I don't focus exclusively on the site of a patient's pain. For starters, pain isn't necessarily a reliable indicator of an injury's source. A heart attack is a great example. You could be having one, and part of your heart could be dying, yet you might not feel much chest pain. Instead, you might feel pain in your arm, jaw, or back. The mind plays an influential role in how we perceive pain and how it manifests. Have you ever seen a kid fall, scrape their knee, and look over at their parents before starting to cry? Or have you noticed that your finger hurts before it even touches a flame? Your brain listens to signals from your body before it creates the sensation of pain.

The disconnect between pain and its source can be further complicated by time. For example, patients often come to see me because of knee pain, but my initial assessment may suggest that the problem actually lies in their feet. The pain in their knees is collateral damage from compensating for other issues, probably over many years. This distinction is crucial, because in this case, treating a patient's knees won't fix their problem.

When I talk about posture, how you stand gives me a sense of where you spend most of your time. If I see your hip hiked up on one side, your pelvis rotated one way, and your shoulder elevated on the other, I will do something you may not expect. I will ask you about your life—what you do, what drives you, and what your hopes and dreams are.

Like a detective trying to piece together clues to solve a mystery, I began working with Nancy twice a week in an attempt to identify a single root cause of her various problems. If I tried something with Nancy and it didn't work, we didn't let it sidetrack us. I'd suggest something else. When we found a technique that did help, we'd keep at it, building on that success in subsequent sessions.

Finally, after two years, Nancy was pain-free and had emptied her medicine cabinet of pills. I pieced together enough clues to resolve the underlying issues that had caused her chronic pain. And as is so often the case, it all began with her posture. Because where there's bad posture, pain and misery are sure to follow.

Futureproofing: The Key to Healthy Longevity

As a physical therapist who oversees a chain of clinics under the brand Myodetox, I've been treating patients like Nancy nearly every day since 2007. During that time, I've encountered hundreds of people crippled by debilitating pain, unclear about what caused it and about how it can be fixed. Many of these patients have seen numerous physical therapists, pain management specialists, and doctors before arriving at my clinic. What I encounter time and again is chronic pain caused by poor posture and a sedentary lifestyle that robs people of their mobility and flexibility and saps their strength. All of these elements feed on and amplify one another. But poor posture lies at the heart of it all. When we address postural issues, pain can resolve and people can move with greater ease and comfort. A vicious cycle becomes a virtuous cycle.

While pain may not be the root cause of your problem, often it's the most pressing manifestation. It may well be the reason you sought out this book. In many respects, we're still in the early stages of understanding the science underlying pain:

how it happens, how it's managed, and hopefully, how it can be stopped. Why does an injury to one part of the body result in pain in another, seemingly unrelated part of the body, as described above? Why is some pain fleeting and some continuous? Unlike bones and organs, the central nervous system can be remodeled by chemical and physical changes. But the science is an abstraction when you're in chronic pain. The pain is all that matters for you in that moment. It has a claustrophobic effect, shrinking the world around you. It's probably making your life a misery, and you want to know how the hell to get rid of it.

Chronic pain isn't the temporary sensation that comes from a stubbed toe or a headache. It's enduring, the continuation of pain long after the original transmitter of that pain is gone. It can become overwhelming, and it can make someone desperate. According to the journal *Progress in Neuro-Psychopharmacology & Biological Psychiatry*, "Individuals with chronic pain are at least twice as likely to report suicidal behaviors or to complete suicide." People on the verge of such a tragic act often live like prisoners in their homes, spending their days on the couch watching TV and popping pain meds, silently mourning lost careers and dead relationships. The prescription medications they rely on can become a health problem in their own right, causing severe side effects and leading to addiction. In the United States alone, thirty-eight people a day, on average, die from an opioid overdose. Many of those tragedies began with prescription pain medicines.

Opioid abuse and addiction have become epidemics because so many people end up hurting, and it's cheaper and easier to get a drug prescription than it is to receive good therapy. Patients shuffle in and out of clinics, looking for relief from their back pain, torn ligaments, pelvic pain, aching shoulders, and other ailments. Back pain is now a billion-dollar industry, with 70 percent of U.S. adults experiencing it at some point during their life. That's why I'm so passionate about these issues, and why I intend to help solve them. I envision a world where back pain isn't a leading growth industry.

Physical therapy, like much of Western medicine, tends to be reactive. The medical system, including physical therapy, focuses on fixing problems rather than preventing them from happening in the first place. Most of the people who land in my office do so in pain. Rather than helping them maximize their full potential, I spend the initial sessions "course-correcting" and simply restoring them to their baseline, which should have been their starting point. Sometimes you have to take one step back to take two steps forward.

I believe optimal alignment and movement patterns will slow down the potential wear and tear from aging. My full-body-treatment approach restores balance by decreasing tension, reducing pain, aligning posture, increasing range of motion, and building strength. I have no doubt that the easier it is for you to line up with gravity, the better you'll breathe, digest, stand, sit, and move.

One of my idols is Bruce Lee, the martial arts icon and movie star. I loved Bruce's disdain for convention, his disregard of boundaries. Unlike his peers, he dabbled in bodybuilding-style workouts and read muscle magazines in search of new workout ideas. I'm similarly curious, open-minded, and unorthodox when it comes to physical therapy. I don't adhere to one school of thought. I pick and choose from among different approaches, combining techniques I like into what works best for my patients while discarding what doesn't.

Traditional physical therapists take a local approach to whatever ails a patient: "Your foot hurts. Let me look at your foot" or "Your knee hurts. Let me look at your knee." My physical therapy approach is holistic, incorporating various strategies, many of which might seem unrelated at first. When patients tell me what's wrong with them, I don't view their complaint, whatever it might be, in isolation. I don't even consider it solely in the context of their whole body. I view it in the context of their life. The wisdom of that approach seems self-evident, but it's surprisingly rare in my field.

Low back pain, neck stiffness, serial headaches—they're all the result of using the body in a way that it wasn't designed for. The modern lifestyle of long work hours, a constant tethering to electronic devices and gadgets, and lack of exercise certainly doesn't help. This lifestyle was ubiquitous before 2020, but for many people, the coronavirus pandemic sent it into overdrive. Suddenly, long work hours became *endless* work hours as the office and the home became one and the same. There was no need to walk down the office hallway to attend a meeting; now you simply had to log into a video conference call.

"Tech neck" and "iHunch" are the sound-bite terms coined to describe forward head posture, where the head tracks forward, out in front of the shoulders, while the eyes remain glued to a device (Figures 1.1, 1.2, 1.3). Fixing these problems entails more than just sitting up straight, but that distills the essence into one essential and straightforward act. Sitting up straight can save people from a lifetime of pain, not to mention surgery and even disability. An ideal posture maintains the natural curves of the neck, middle back, and lower back. In contrast, a slouching posture places great stress on the muscles of the back and neck, as well as on the spine itself. It also contributes to depression, chronic fatigue, and chronic pain. When you slouch every day, your spine is like a door that doesn't fit properly in a doorjamb. Open an ill-fitting door over many years, and the wear and tear will be far greater than if the door swung the way it should.

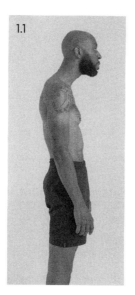 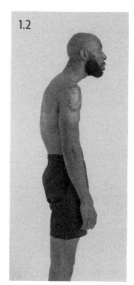 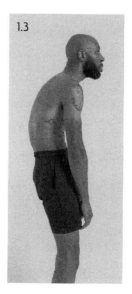

Progression of "tech neck": head forward posture, head forward posture with shoulders rounding, head forward posture with shoulders mid back rounding

DO THIS NOW: Dial in your work-from-home setup. Myodetox saw a 50 percent bump in patients with posture-related back and neck pain during the coronavirus pandemic. Many of these patients had switched from working in an office to working from home. At work, they often had help setting up an ergonomically sound workspace. At home, they were on their own. Home offices tend to be a mishmash of whatever is available to work on. Some of us are lucky enough to have a dedicated space for a proper work-from-home setup, while others end up on the floor with their laptop. Whatever your situation, use these guidelines to set up your area (Figure 1.4):

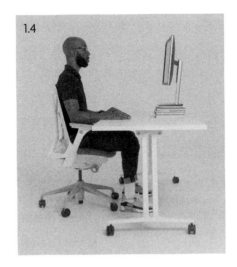

1.4

Proper sitting posture

▷ Keep your screen as close to eye level as possible. Stacking books under your monitor can be a huge help.

▷ Keep your keyboard at a comfortable distance from your body, allowing for a 90-degree bend in your elbows.

▷ When typing, keep your wrists off the table (active) instead of leaving them on it (passive). Resting your wrists occasionally is okay, but prolonged pressure on your wrists can irritate sensitive nerves and tendons.

▷ Keep your knees and hips bent at around 90 degrees.

▷ Get up and move every half hour. Doing the movement exercises found later in this book will help keep your joints and muscles from stiffening.

Break Glass When Needed!

QUICK-FIX POSTURE FIX

If you find that you've been hunched for any length of time, the shoulder blade squeeze, aka scapular retraction, is a simple way to reset your posture:

1. Let your arms hang down by your sides (Figure 1.5).

2. Slightly round your shoulders (Figure 1.6).

3. Pull your shoulder blades back toward your spine and down (Figure 1.7).

4. I typically tell patients to do that motion ten to twenty times per session.

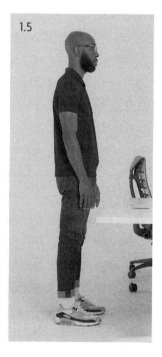
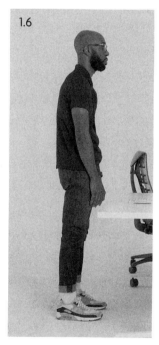
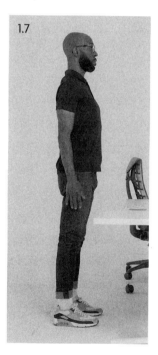

I want you to do it every hour as part of your sitting breaks. This stretch can even be done while you're waiting at a red light or stuck in traffic. This movement gets the blood flowing to those muscles, but more important, it's a reminder to get your shoulder blades back and into their proper position.

When someone slouches for hours at a time, pressure increases on certain areas of their spine. This can work for a while. But there's a limit to how much the spine can handle in such a compromised position, and once damaged, the spine will never be quite the same. It's so intricate and multifaceted in how it's constructed that it's hard, if not impossible, to repair perfectly.

Don't get me wrong, sitting is not inherently bad. To suggest otherwise would be ridiculous. When sitting happens in short bouts, with the body in a biomechanically sound position, it's fine from a musculoskeletal standpoint. The problem is the protracted lengths of time people spend sitting and their tendency to sit in one position without switching it up, as well as the forces these habits, working in tandem, place on the spine. The answer isn't standing all day, either; standing for too long also causes problems, which I'll discuss in more detail later. Still, I believe changing your life begins with something as easy as sitting well 80 percent of the time you're sitting. I'm convinced it's the crucial first step for physical and mental well-being.

DO THIS NOW: Try sitting on a resistance ball at your desk (Figure 1.8). It's tough to slouch on an exercise ball without having it fly out from under you, dumping you on your behind. The ball forces you to maintain a decent posture while activating your core to stabilize your body. Sitting on a ball is sometimes hailed as a way to burn a few extra calories, but "few" is the operative word. The greater benefit is how it forces you to stay mindful of what you're doing and sit up straight.

If you don't have a resistance ball handy, sitting on the edge of your seat with your knees at roughly 90 degrees and your feet flat will automatically make it easier for you to sit up straight. Slouching with your feet flat on the floor is really uncomfortable.

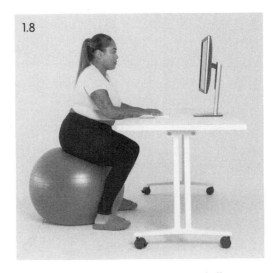

1.8

Sitting posture on an exercise ball

What Your Posture Is Saying to the World

Each of the body's joints plays a role in maintaining posture and balance, whether you're standing, performing an action, or recovering after a misstep. Without well-developed postural muscles to counter the forces of gravity, the human body would be little more than a bag of bones. Most of us grow up blissfully unaware of our posture until one day a teacher admonishes us for sliding down at our desk or a parent reprimands us for reclining at the dining table. When you are a kid, being scolded about posture feels punitive, not to mention pointless. Who cares how you sit if that's what feels comfortable? As a result, commands to sit up straight go in one ear and out the other.

Here's why good posture is crucial. For starters, it conveys strength and dominance, while slouching conveys weakness and submission. The importance of posture is evident as far back as antiquity; in Greek statues, subjects stand tall even while twisting or striding. These are commanding figures, human beings with the aura of gods. When ancient artists sought to immortalize the human form, they showed it at its best, not wincing and mouthing, "Ouch, my back!" History commemorates winners, and winners stand straight and tall.

We tend to think of poor posture from a sedentary lifestyle as being a recent phenomenon, but there is historical precedent for allowing sloth to induce bad habits. In ancient Egypt's hieroglyphics, for example, the laborers are pictured with textbook posture: back straight, head up, perfectly balanced. Often the people being pictured carry a load above their head. If they were hunched over or had forward head lean, their loads would have tumbled to the ground.

Equally telling are depictions of the royals and ruling class. Many exhibit slouched posture or forward head lean of the sort you might see today from a twentysomething with tech neck. Presumably, the elites of antiquity were couch potatoes compared to the laborers, and their bodies were already paying the sort of postural price we see everywhere today.

In the wild, posture also sends a message. When two wolves come face-to-face, for example, the dominant one remains upright, while the submissive one flattens its body and grovels—a stance that also happens to help shield it from attack. This sort of phenomenon occurs throughout the animal kingdom, often as a way of *avoiding*, rather than instigating, conflict. "Don't mess with me, for your own good," is the message being delivered. Avoiding conflict enables the potential combatants to focus on more important matters like finding food.

DO THIS NOW: Assess your inside—and see how it manifests on the outside. How's your mood? Did you wake up this morning ready to conquer the day? If so, you may be standing straight and proudly. Do you feel overwhelmed? You may be holding tension in your neck and shoulder girdle. Do you feel sad? You're likely looking downward, with your shoulders rolled inward and your rib cage collapsed. Just as is true in the wild, your posture telegraphs your emotions.

The body language of humans is equally telling. Next time you're in a bar, look at the posture of the other patrons. The slouching person is usually off in a corner, sipping a drink and jabbing at their cell phone, pretending to be busy and preoccupied, their protective posture a shield deployed against rejection. At the center of attention are those who stand up straight; they have gravitational pull, and others settle comfortably into their orbit. Unspoken messages are being sent by everyone in such settings.

Better to develop an awareness of your posture sooner than later. Poor posture afflicts people of all ages, but it tends to worsen with age—and by 2050, one in six people worldwide will be over age sixty-five. This spells trouble, as the high cost of inactivity is compounded by physical deficits that pile up over time.

A great misconception about good posture is that maintaining it is hard work, an endurance test of sorts. On the contrary, good posture should be effortless, with no sensation of "doing" or "holding." It's about gently organizing your bones, relaxing, getting grounded, softening the muscles around the pelvis and shoulders, and feeling the length of your body.

Animals have hardwired behavioral traits that come standard issue with their species, in the same way a particular car model has factory-installed features. Animals operate primarily on instinct, regardless of where and under what circumstances they're born. Humans, however, develop based on the environment they grow up in and what they're taught. They learn from experience. For example, Vietnamese parents raised me in a French-Canadian city, Montreal. Growing up, I learned Vietnamese in our household, French in school, and English from watching *Sesame Street*. This melting pot of languages and experiences helped define my speech patterns. But even though I spent twenty-plus years speaking French, ever since I moved to Toronto and stopped using French daily, I've struggled to find words when speaking it with others. No matter how deeply ingrained the pattern, it still must be continuously reinforced with experience.

Just as with languages and speech patterns, how you sit and stand also reflects your experiences. If you have a particular way of moving or sitting, it can be undone or improved if you're unhappy with it. Your body needs to be exposed to a different movement experience for it to transform into something else.

An old teacher of mine used to say that your story is written in your structure. He meant that in the same way your personality is a reflection of your various life experiences to date, your "posture personality" is shaped by everything your body has been exposed to up to this point, reinforced by habit. This "personality" is an accumulation of your memory and experiences.

Postural decline isn't an inevitable part of aging, but avoiding it takes work. Your body can move effectively and efficiently throughout your adulthood if you take care of it with the posture hygiene routine outlined in this book. This routine can help futureproof your body and reverse the clock on aging. If that sounds impossible, it's not. You have a fixed chronological age that begins with the date on your birth certificate. It can't be changed. But your body also has a structural age, which is actually a more accurate and more telling measure of longevity, I would argue. That age, you *can* alter.

There's an expression, "So-and-so is seventy but has the body of a forty-year-old!" That's what I'm talking about here. The reverse is true: An inactive twenty-year-old can have the structural age of someone in their forties. The most extreme example might be a smoker. They add decades to their actual age because of one harmful habit. Smoking doesn't just age their lungs prematurely; it poisons the body at a cellular level, which is why it often causes cancer.

What's more, the older you are, the harder it becomes to undo the damage wrought by many years of poor posture. If you've been hunching your whole life and try to address postural issues in your fifties, the amount of damage you can undo may be limited. If you're in your twenties or thirties, the damage may be reversible. In either case, it's better to prevent the damage in the first place.

There's a genetic aspect to the human spine that can influence posture throughout someone's life. Yet where posture is concerned, for most people, nurture trumps nature. How you sit and stand today is a product of the life choices you've made along the way. Maybe you hunch as an adult because you were shy when you were younger and wanted to blend in rather than stand out. There are a million potential reasons why you might be slouching today.

Rather than discouraging me, this realization gives me hope, and it should give *you* hope, too. Once you become aware of which forces shaped your current posture, you can take action. And that's what's fascinating about posture. In many ways, even if we don't realize it, our posture is the best reflection of our life experiences to date. So if you want to improve your life, start by changing your posture.

2 THE BLUEPRINT OF YOUR BODY'S POSTURE

YOU CAN'T DISCUSS POSTURE without understanding the spine—the human body's central support structure—and the pelvis. Let's start with the spine. This structure must be incredibly strong to support your body, yet extremely flexible, too, allowing for all sorts of movement, which is why your backbone isn't straight like a ruler. The spine's trademark curves, which you'll read about a lot in this book, help distribute mechanical stress during movement, in the same way that a bridge needs to absorb all sorts of stress (wind, trucks, etc.) yet never fails to hold.

Unfortunately, the spine is also one of the most common sources of pain in the human body. Because the spine is involved in nearly every human activity, back pain makes itself known no matter what you do, even when you're just shifting your weight. One reason the spine is a bony fortress is to protect the vital nerves traveling down it. Lower down in the spine is where you get more of the chronic type of pain, as those discs and vertebrae are prone to wear and tear from poor sitting, bad posture, and careless lifting.

The spine comprises twenty-four small bones called vertebrae; stacked like building blocks, they form the spinal canal. The canal's primary purpose is to shield the spinal cord and nerves from injury. This is of paramount importance because the spinal cord transmits messages of sensation and movement back and forth between the brain and the body. The stacked vertebrae are separated by small "cushions" called discs. These discs are filled with a gel-like material, kind of like the filling in a jelly doughnut. The spine discs act as miniature shock absorbers; along with protecting the spine, they allow for mobility. (Without them, you'd be as stiff as a board.) When the spine is subjected to repeated stress in the form of compression and twisting, small tears show up in the area surrounding the "jelly" center of the disc. Eventually that soft center can be pushed out of its space, a troublesome event called a herniation. The "jelly" that's pushed out can end up pressing against nerves, causing intense pain, tingling, numbness, and in extreme cases even loss of strength and movement in the affected area.

The vertebrae and discs are connected by what are called facet joints. Ligaments connect the spine to the rest of the body, holding the whole complex together.

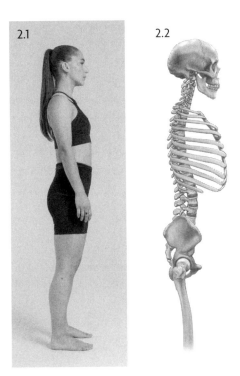

Well-balanced posture viewed from the side. Note the S shape.

The spine should run straight down when viewed from behind. Viewed from the right side, it should resemble the shape of the letter S (Figures 2.1, 2.2). The three sections of the spine—cervical (upper), thoracic (middle), and lumbar (lower)—each have a distinctive, gently sloping curve. The cervical spine (in the neck area) curves slightly inward, like a backward C; whereas the thoracic spine (T-spine for short) curves outward, like a regular C. The lumbar spine, like the cervical spine, curves inward, also like a backward C.

However, some people have abnormalities of the spine that can stem from postural habits and genetics, including:

LORDOSIS: The lower spine curves too far inward, like someone just poked the person in the back with a stick (Figures 2.3, 2.4).

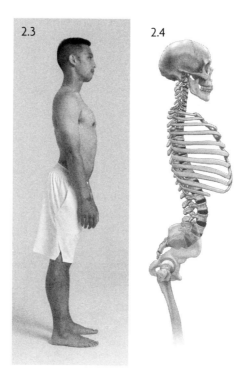

2.3   2.4

KYPHOSIS: The middle spine flexes forward excessively. An exaggerated example of this excessive rounding would be the Hunchback of Notre Dame (Figures 2.5, 2.6).

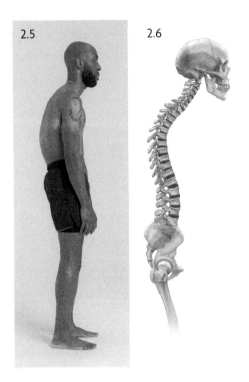

2.5   2.6

FLAT BACK: Instead of the lower back curving inward too much, it doesn't curve enough, straightening the bottom of the S shape (Figures 2.7, 2.8). This condition can make it much more difficult for someone to stand up for any length of time.

SCOLIOSIS: This condition involves a sideways curve to the spine when viewed from behind (Figure 2.9). Congenital scoliosis is the most common spinal deformity. The vertebrae don't form and stack properly in the womb.

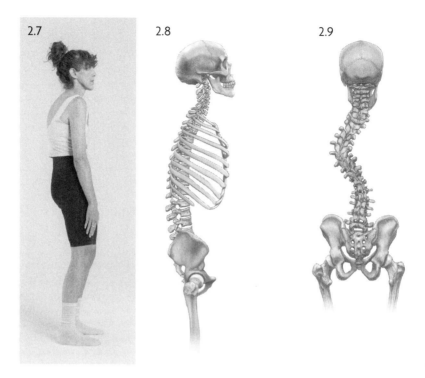

All three of the major spine segments (cervical, thoracic, and lumbar) participate in all sorts of daily activities. Every time you move your head and neck, your
cervical spine is involved. Every time you rotate your torso, your thoracic spine is
working. Every time you bend over to pick up an object or tie your shoelaces, your
lumbar spine is at play. The more hypermobile a spinal segment is, the more prone it
is to damage from misalignment and poor movement habits. When you have limited
mobility in one area of your body, your brain will compensate by recruiting another
area to get the job done.

But this takes a toll over time. I'll give you an example. Say you're an avid golfer,
but, for whatever reason, your thoracic spine isn't as mobile as it should be. When
you tee off, your healthy lumbar spine has to compensate for the stiff thoracic spine
slacking off above it. Fast-forward a few years, and suddenly your lumbar spine is
jacked up, too.

Here is a list of just some of the daily stressors affecting each spine segment:

CERVICAL SPINE MOVEMENTS

► Rotating your head while driving

► Bending your neck when looking at your phone

► Holding up your head while working at a desk

► Sleeping with your neck bent backward or turned

THORACIC SPINE MOVEMENTS

► Playing sports (e.g., golf, boxing, tennis, baseball) that rely heavily on torso rotation

► Rotating your body because of your office setup (e.g., the computer may be oriented to your right or left)

► Hunching while sitting

► Hunching because you're too tall, so you need to bend over to speak to someone eye to eye

► Sleeping in a twisted position

LUMBAR SPINE MOVEMENTS

▶ Hunching while sitting

▶ Leaning to one side while sitting and standing

▶ Using poor mechanics with lifts (e.g., lifting with your back without the help of your legs. Figures 2.10 and 2.11 demonstrate good versus poor lifting)

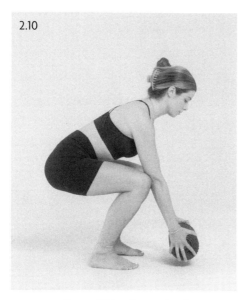
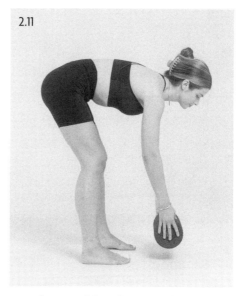

Proper lifting form using legs   *Improper lifting form using back*

▶ Rotating/twisting your back with excessive load

▶ Sleeping in positions not favorable to your back

▶ Being employed in certain types of jobs: construction; employment that involves standing all day (e.g., factory workers, restaurant servers) or sitting all day (e.g., office workers, truck drivers, gig economy drivers)

▶ Walking and running with poor mechanics

The pelvis comprises three bones: the sacrum flanked by an ilium bone on either side, together forming a closed ring. It's a container for various organs; in fact, the word "pelvis" comes from the Greek *pella*, meaning "bowl." This basin happens to be jammed full of the human body's reproductive organs, so it's precious and sensitive real estate. The pelvis also serves as an anchor point for many muscles, both small and large, as well as our center of gravity. It has a significant impact on posture, movement, and function. Any pelvic imbalances inevitably will show up in posture and movement, often leading to pain as well.

The hip flexors and extensors have a lot to do with pelvic alignment, but three compartments of the leg also affect the pelvis: the anterior (front), medial (middle), and posterior (back) compartments. The main muscles involved with the anterior compartment are the quadriceps. The medial compartment muscles are the adductor (groin) muscles, and the posterior compartment contains the hamstring muscles. Any imbalance in one compartment can lead to overuse, weakness, or tightness in the other.

"Pelvic tilt" is a term physical therapists and others use to describe the position of the pelvis relative to the thighbones and the rest of the body. Your pelvis can tilt forward, backward, or to either side. Usually, if one pelvic bone is tilted, say, forward, the other pelvic bone will be tilted forward as well, and the same goes for backward tilts. However, sometimes the two pelvic bones can tilt in opposite directions: one forward, one backward. Among other issues, this can lead to one leg appearing longer than the other to the naked eye, even though it's not. Pelvic tilts are further discussed in chapters 6 through 9.

The Ups and Downs of Sitting and Standing

I'm going to write at length in this book about the many problems caused by sedentary behavior, particularly lengthy stretches spent slouching behind a desk. But before we get into how *not* to stand and sit, let's talk about how you *should* stand and sit.

I'll start with standing posture, because how you stand will greatly impact how you sit. This is the ideal standing posture (Figure 2.12):

▶ Ears aligned over shoulders

▶ Shoulders aligned above hips

▶ Neutral pelvic position

▶ Knees soft; no locking or hyperextension

▶ The three natural S curves in the spine maintained but not exaggerated

▶ Feet hip-width apart

▶ Feet pointed straight ahead, not splayed outward like a duck or inward like a pigeon. Weight should be distributed evenly through both feet, in a tripod position.

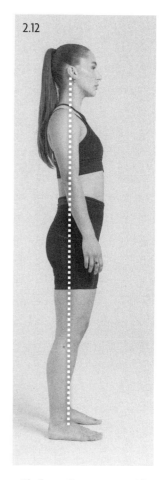

2.12

Many people have poor standing posture, especially when they're anchored in one place for any time. (This is why standing desks aren't the antidote for too much sitting. The pressure on the spine when sitting versus standing is pretty similar.) It doesn't take that long for a person's standing posture to disintegrate, and it's usually the positioning of the pelvis that gives way first, either by tilting or shifting. Most people naturally favor one side of their body when standing, and they lean into the hip on that side. Shifting the pelvis by leaning in either direction changes your posture, usually in ways that place pressure on your spine.

Ideal standing posture with the white line highlighting balance straight through

DO THIS NOW: When standing while working at a computer, place one foot on a stool or on some books (Figures 2.13, 2.14). This will automatically balance your pelvis and prevent you from going into hip hike. Make sure to do this with both legs, five minutes at a time as needed.

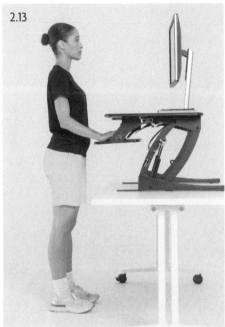

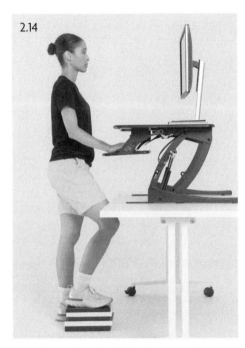

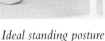

Ideal standing posture   *Foot elevated with books or stool*

One school of thought maintains that since standing is not sitting, ipso facto, standing must be good for you. But scant evidence suggests that standing at your desk in and of itself (as opposed to sitting) offers much in the way of health benefits. You'll often hear how standing at a desk turns a body into a fat-burning machine, but I've seen a few studies where they've compared the energy expended by those who are sitting compared to those who are standing, and there's not much difference.

Another reason standing in the same spot for long stretches isn't that much better than sitting for long periods is the impact on cognitive function. One study found that people who stood at their desks for two hours actually got worse at certain

---

How Much Time Should Be Spent Sitting Versus Standing?

The traditional work model calls for people to work for eight hours, and employees are often encouraged to get up at least once every hour. However, there's a school of thought that advocates getting up and standing for at least *half* the time you're at work. Assuming an eight-hour workday, that's four hours of standing—truly a tall order, especially if performed without a break! Another way to skin the cat would be to alternate sitting and standing in thirty-minute intervals. Again, that's no easy task, but a goal worth striving for. If this isn't possible (and for many, it would be difficult), aim to limit sitting to at most thirty minutes at a time. If the timer on your smartphone or smart watch says you're approaching thirty minutes "in the cockpit," get up, walk around, and do some of the exercises in this book. Your body will thank you.

As for the sitting postures discussed below, the obvious point to make is that if you're going to sit for thirty minutes, you should attempt to do so in the "military sitting" position and lounge position (Figures 2.20, 2.21). Other poorer positions are inevitable, but they should be minimized to, at most, five to ten minutes in an hour.

---

cognitive functions, including problem-solving. Marketers of standing desks claim they will increase your productivity at work, but I've seen nothing to support that notion.

There's a general lack of awareness among workers regarding how they sit. And researchers have found that the more concentration and focus desk work requires— and the more stress desk workers are under—the less aware they are of their posture.

When you sit slouched, the front of your pelvis will tilt backward, which will flatten your lumbar spine, placing increased pressure on your spine. In light of that reality, this is the ideal sitting posture (Figure 2.15):

▶ Feet flat on the floor

▶ Knees at 90-degree angles

▶ Hips at 90-degree angles and in line with your lumbar spine and shoulders

▶ Back flush with the back of the chair

- ► Solid lumbar support in the back of your chair

- ► Shoulders in line with your lumbar spine

- ► Arms loose but supported

- ► Elbows at 90-degree angles

- ► Eyes anywhere from midway up the monitor to the upper third

- ► No side leaning for any length of time

- ► Use a stool if your feet don't touch the floor

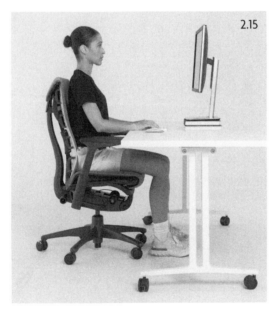

Keeping the elbows at 90-degree angles is essential yet often overlooked. If the elbows are any higher, the trapezius muscles kick in to raise the arms high enough for the hands to reach the keyboard. Eventually this will lead to fatigue and muscle spasms.

I want to stress that this is an idealized and aspirational version of the perfect sitting form. I don't expect you to sit like this all the time, unless you're a robot. You may have heard of the so-called 80/20 rule in nutrition, which states that if you eat "clean" 80 percent of the time, you can indulge in junk food and desserts 20 percent of the time while still making progress toward your goals. I'm asking you to apply that same 80/20 ratio to your sitting posture: Aim to sit "correctly," as described above, 80 percent of the time. Hit that target, and I'm fine if you slouch or sit however you want the other 20 percent. It's a good thing to switch it up rather than sitting with a rigid posture all the time—even sitting with an ideal posture. Just as your taste buds grow weary of eating the same foods all the time, it's essential to vary your sitting positions.

DO THIS NOW: Grab a twelve- or sixteen-ounce water bottle and place it between your back and your chair (Figures 2.16, 2.17, 2.18). Every ten minutes or whenever you feel comfortable—whichever comes first—switch the position of the water bottle. This will help you support your spine and teach you how to use different muscles to support yourself.

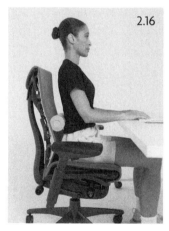
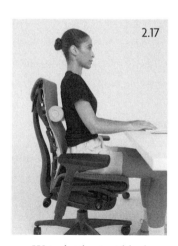
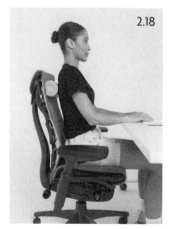

Water bottle at low back	*Water bottle at mid back*	*Water bottle at upper back*

Instead of thinking that there's a "good" way of sitting all the time and a "bad" way of sitting all the time, think of sitting postures as falling along a continuum, sort of like the pain scale at the doctor's office, where the face is smiling and happy at one end and in agony and tears at the other. On the sitting continuum, the far left is slouching, which turns off the muscle activity customarily used to support good posture. Support is left up to the spine, ligaments, and joints instead of the muscles designed to support you. Slouching some of the time is an acceptable part of the 20 percent, but don't exceed that percentage.

Over at the far right is the neutral and supportive sitting position described above as the ideal, in which muscles support your posture and protect your body from stress. Aim for this better posture 80 percent of the time, knowing that if someone were to measure the angles of your elbows and knees, you wouldn't be perfect nearly that often. But over time, you can approach perfection.

Most people's sitting falls somewhere in between those two poles of slouching and sitting up straight. The farther to the right your sitting is at a given moment, the better off you'll be.

DO THIS NOW: Don't over-rely on sitting or standing for work. The key to better health isn't to replace sitting with standing, or vice versa. It's to break up sitting or standing. One helpful strategy is to get up and move as much as you can. Challenge yourself to move for at least 25 percent of your day.

Common Sitting Postures and Their Implications

SUPER SLOUCH

Super slouch (Figure 2.19) is commonly seen in individuals who might be hyperfocused on a task, completing work under excessive stress, and generally fatigued (I'm super slouching as I edit this book on a thirteen-inch computer screen). Take note that commonly, people may assume this position if they're having visual problems. So I suggest getting your eyes checked if you think that may be an issue.

ADVANTAGES: Decreased energy expenditure, good for resting muscles, may allow for increased focus.

DISADVANTAGES: Stresses the entire spinal column and pelvis; increases tightness to the posterior chain of the back; compresses trunk in the front.

DURATION: Five minutes at a time, max! Don't absentmindedly get stuck in this position.

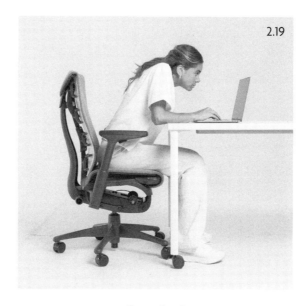

2.19

Super slouch

MILITARY SITTING

Military sitting (Figure 2.20) is hard to maintain at first, but if you practice it will become easier and easier over time. It's the ideal posture to practice if your job requires you to sit long hours staring at a screen. Once this position becomes easy for you to slip in and out of, you'll know that your postural muscles are strong.

ADVANTAGES: Projects confidence, balanced stress to the body, improved breathing, postural strength training.

DISADVANTAGES: Effortful, requires training, initially may feel uncomfortable.

DURATION: Thirty minutes at a time.

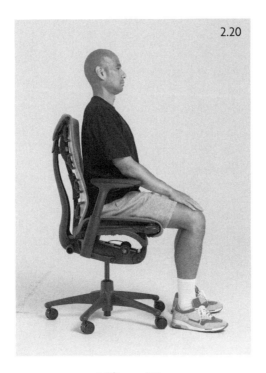

2.20

Military sitting

LOUNGE SITTING

Lounge sitting (Figure 2.21) is the more relaxed style of sitting that we're likely to favor if we're reading, or entering a flow state while working. Either way, this sitting facilitates a state of relaxation, which many of us strive for. More important, lounge sitting mitigates the negatives of slouching.

ADVANTAGES: At a 135-degree angle, the least amount of stress to the spinal discs. Also facilitates a relaxed posture, whether for working or zoning out.

DISADVANTAGE: Most chairs don't support this position while working, and your postural muscles will suffer the longer you indulge.

DURATION: Thirty minutes at a time.

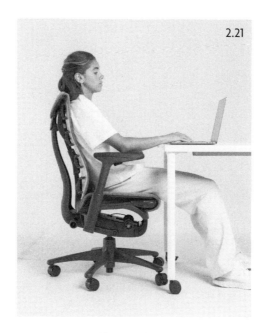

Lounge sitting

OFFICE TABLE LEAN

The office table lean (Figure 2.22) is a compromise between the military posture and the super slouch position. In this position you hinge at your waist while maintaining an upright trunk—notice the shoulders don't round. This shows that you're focused on your task and somewhat aware of your posture. The downside? There's still a head forward posture, and you place a lot of weight on your arms.

ADVANTAGES: Hinge position challenges the postural muscles. It's the compromise between military sitting and super slouching.

DISADVANTAGES: If your postural muscles aren't trained to be strong, you'll round at your low back and increase forward head posture.

DURATION: Ten minutes at a time. Aim for less, unless used as a stretch.

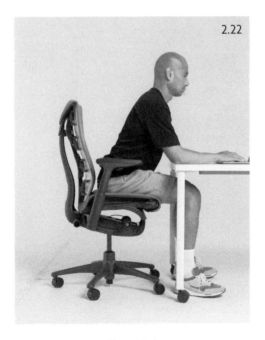

Office table lean

CORNER-OF-THE-COUCH LEAN

The corner-of-the-couch lean (Figure 22.3) is most likely the position you choose if you're watching TV. Though it's meant to be a relaxing position, my issue with it is that too much time spent leaning and sinking your weight into one side eventually leads to an imbalance in your body. If you have a tendency to lean toward one side, try using this position as a stretch by leaning toward the other side for ten minutes.

ADVANTAGES: Opens space on one side and facilitates relaxation. Also helpful: Support from the couch alleviates the need for the body to support itself.

DISADVANTAGES: Asymmetrical posture stresses the spine and musculature of the hips and back.

DURATION: Ten minutes at a time. Aim for less.

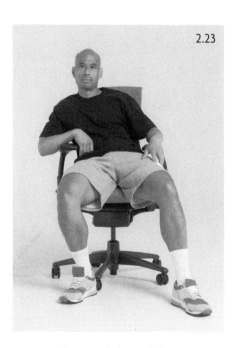

2.23

Corner-of-the-couch lean

HIP STRETCH POSE

Many people assume the hip stretch pose (Figure 2.24) if they want to naturally stretch one hip, especially when they're looking to get comfortable (e.g., during a stressful meeting). My issue is that people tend to focus on the same hip, and this leads to a shift in weight to the side being stretched.

ADVANTAGES: Shifts weight while maintaining a modified military sitting posture, and stretches the posterior hip.

DISADVANTAGES: Asymmetrical stress to the pelvis and sides of the hip joint. People also tend to focus on one hip, and not switch between left and right evenly.

DURATION: Ten minutes at a time. Aim to switch legs after a few minutes, if possible.

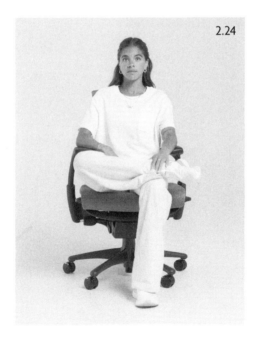

2.24

Hip stretch pose

CROSS-LEG POSE

This is definitely the pose (Figure 2.25) my mom struck when I got in trouble as a kid. It's upright but intimidating. Truthfully, it requires significant range of motion at the hip to perform, so not everyone can do this one. Like the hip stretch pose, the cross-leg pose facilitates good posture while being energy efficient, but I would suggest switching legs equally to minimize imbalances.

ADVANTAGES: Facilitates the natural and correct curvature of the upper and lower back.

DISADVANTAGES: Asymmetrical stress on the pelvis, and the front of the hip that joins the top leg will be pinched (joint, capsule, and labrum). Also, using one leg exclusively will lead to an imbalance.

DURATION: Ten minutes at a time. Aim to switch legs after a few minutes, if possible.

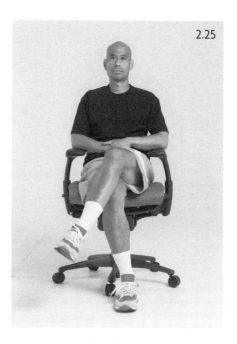

Cross-leg pose

FORWARD LEAN (CONFIDENT GAMER POSE)

I love this posture (Figure 2.26), but maybe not for the right reasons. It's the one video gamers often adopt when staring at their TV. It represents someone hyperfocused. (Hint: If someone in your class sits like this, you want that person in your study group.) The downside? It facilitates a chin poke, and therefore leads to the head forward posture. You'll round out your low and mid back within minutes.

ADVANTAGES: Facilitates focus on a task and rest from the upright posture.

DISADVANTAGES: It'll eventually lead to a head forward posture, and it may signal visual problems.

DURATION: Ten minutes at a time. Aim for less.

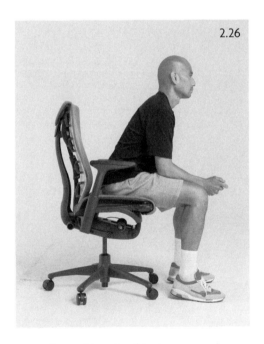

Forward lean (confident gamer pose)

STRESSED-OUT GAMER

The stressed-out gamer posture (Figure 2.27) feels a little personal to me. In physical therapy school, I remember slipping into this pose while listening to lectures on cardiovascular medicine—a worthy topic that just didn't come naturally to me. My anxiety had me hinging forward with an excessive head forward posture. Basically, I was stressed. But this posture can also be observed in someone who's really *into* what's in front of them!

ADVANTAGES: Facilitates focus.

DISADVANTAGES: Rounded low back, mid back, and neck with an excessive head forward posture. Moreover, this position combined with stress is a poor mix for your overall posture.

DURATION: Five minutes, max. Ideally, never.

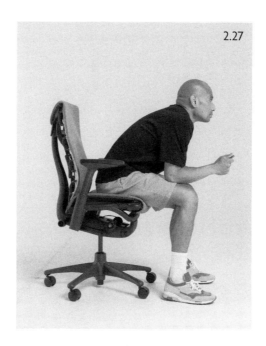

2.27

Stressed-out gamer

There are exceptions to these sitting guidelines that kick in when someone has structural issues such as unusually long or short legs, wide hips, asymmetrical spinal curves, or pain. For example, someone who's tall and has long tibias may sit with knees higher than hips, placing the body in a position of perpetual lumbar spine flexion. The knees and hips should be aligned, so the solution is to elevate the hips with a pillow.

Yoga has a lot to teach us about sitting positions and their effects on us. How we sit at a given moment speaks volumes about our emotions. You can tell when someone is tense because they develop a guarded posture, often crossing their arms and legs. The tension is almost palpable. Conversely, you can tell when someone is relaxed and happy because their posture tends to be open, welcoming, comfortable, at ease, like they're at a summer barbecue and don't have a care in the world. These postures tend to be self-perpetuating, too. You won't go from tense to relaxed until you uncross your arms and legs and start breathing more calmly and deeply, rather than with short, staccato breaths.

Recognizing the effect different positions have on the mind, body, and spirit, yoga teaches its practitioners how to assume positions that reinforce positivity. It's all about developing an awareness of the relationship between your feelings and your posture. The next time you receive praise at work, take note of how you're sitting immediately afterward. You're likely to be upright and alert, not slouched. The next time you're criticized or reprimanded, do the same self-inspection. Chances are you'll be slouching as if you are about to slide under the desk. By assuming the posture you naturally adopt when you're feeling good, you can make yourself feel good even in the absence of praise. Likewise, when you slouch, it can have the effect of making you feel bad even in the absence of criticism.

Break Glass When Needed!

QUICK-FIX HIP STRETCH

A tiny muscle you've probably never heard of has a powerful effect on your daily movements. It's called the piriformis, and when it's healthy, it allows you to move your hips freely, thus reducing the strain on your lower back. Unfortunately, your piriformis is probably tight if you spend much of your day staring at a screen. This tightness usually leads to discomfort in your hips and low back.

To counteract this tightness, here's a simple stretch you can perform without even leaving your chair:

1. Start by crossing your legs, so one foot and ankle rests on the other knee.

2. Sit up tall and place one hand on your knee and the other on your foot (Figure 2.28).

3. Keeping your spine straight, bend your upper body toward your hips, leading with your chest (Figure 2.29).

4. Apply gentle pressure to your crossed knee to feel a stretch in the hips and the lower back of the bent leg (Figure 2.30).

5. Be sure not to forward flex your neck.

6. Hold for thirty seconds.

7. Do three reps per side.

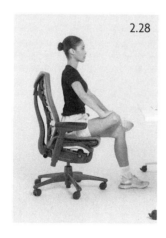
2.28

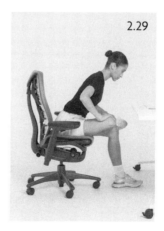
2.29

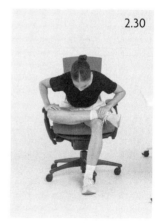
2.30

Sedentary Is the New Smoking

Health threats often emerge suddenly, like when you round a bend on a trail and come face-to-face with a predator. A new virus that sweeps across the globe also comes to mind. But often it takes years, even decades, for something once thought harmless to be unmasked for what it is: a public health menace.

In the first half of the twentieth century, smoking was viewed as a harmless pastime. Many thought cigarettes were not only glamorous but healthy, just as sugary sodas were initially marketed to an unsuspecting public as a health tonic and energy booster. Even as lung cancer rates began rising along with tobacco use, experts were slow to connect smoking with cancer. Not until the 1950s did researchers persuasively link them, and it took another decade or two for the public to begin rejecting the smoking habit.

Sedentary behavior, another activity that might seem harmless at first glance, has emerged as a public health issue in the early twenty-first century. A study published in *The Lancet* estimated the costs of a sedentary lifestyle at $67.5 billion a year worldwide. Mind you, that was before a pandemic forced people inside, shut down gyms, and drastically curtailed social interaction for more than a year.

DO THIS NOW: Break the rules—take your next Zoom call on a walk. The rules changed when everyone started working from home more. You're expected to take back-to-back meetings, solving problems while slumped in the same spot on the couch hour after hour. Ever wonder why your brain gets in a rut as you deepen the grooves in your couch? It's because you're not moving. Do yourself a favor and try to solve the next problem while taking a walk. You'll be surprised how much sharper and more inspired your brain will be.

Sedentary behavior often involves sitting. Mind you, as I mentioned before, sitting isn't inherently bad. The problem is that large numbers of people sit too often, for too long at a time, and with poor posture, often while performing a desk job.

According to the Centers for Disease Control and Prevention (CDC), one in four Americans sits for more than eight hours a day. Not coincidentally, that's the length of a standard workday, and many people sit nearly the entire time they're working.

The perils of excessive sitting first became apparent to public health experts when researchers shared the results of a study comparing transit drivers, who sat behind a wheel all day, with conductors and guards who spent more time on their feet. As it turns out, the sedentary transit drivers were twice as likely as the conductors and guards to develop heart disease.

Can exercise undo the damage wrought by lengthy sitting? Potentially . . . if you're willing to do moderate-intensity physical activity for sixty to seventy-five minutes every day. In a meta-analysis of more than 1 million people published in 2016, that's how much exercise it took to offset the increased death risk from sitting for more than eight hours a day.

The human body isn't designed to stand or sit in one position for too long. Yet so many people across the globe have never been so inactive. That's worrisome because of the strong correlation between sedentary behaviors, such as sitting, and many causes of death, particularly heart disease and type 2 diabetes, the twin lifestyle-disease killers. In fact, 6 percent of all deaths worldwide can be attributed to inactivity, as can significant percentages of all cases of breast and colon cancers, type 2 diabetes, and heart disease.

DO THIS NOW: Get up and move every thirty minutes. Move around for three to five minutes on these micro-breaks. This might be unrealistic for certain people due to the nature of their job, but these breaks should be doable for most people. It can be as simple as going for a brief walk. It gives those postural muscles a break so they can reset and start over. Why thirty minutes? Any less than that, and it may be hard to stay in a groove at work. Any more than that, and you're getting too comfortable in an inactive position—which will feel uncomfortable when you finally move again. Most of the current research suggests thirty minutes as the cutoff point when you need to move around or change something.

Modern societies have increasingly engineered physical activity out of everyday life, from transportation to work to leisure time. In particular, computers, smartphones, and other electronic devices have ushered in what might be called the Sedentary Age. Human progress has witnessed countless inventions that have lowered the cost of moving inefficiently. Those who would have become prey for some beast in ancient times can now turn a key and drive to their destination. If you can't climb a stairwell, no worries—take an escalator or an elevator. It's our physical evolution occurring in reverse: While the human brain has grown bigger and more intelligent, our bodies have grown weaker and less mobile.

We live in a world of people who experience life through a phone yet are wholly out of touch with their body, mind, and spirit. On average teens use their smartphone for nearly seven and a half hours a day. You don't need a statistician to tell you how addicted people are to their phones, though. Next time you're at the doctor's office or waiting for your car to be repaired, look around. Don't worry about appearing nosy or obtrusive; your attention will go unnoticed. Your fellow patrons will be slumped where they sit, staring or jabbing at an electronic device. I even see this at parties where the whole point is to interact face-to-face with others who are present! No wonder so many people have neck and back pain.

The iHunch trend shows no signs of abating. On the contrary, it's easy to envision a future in which human bodies are little more than host organisms for increasingly sophisticated and addictive electronics. People worry about robots taking over eventually, but how different would that future be from the present? Maybe we're already well into the process, albeit unwittingly.

When it comes to electronic devices and poor posture, computers and smartphones garner most of the attention, but tablets such as the iPad pose unique challenges. Because the tablet is relatively small and portable, people use them in all sorts of different positions, including lying in bed or on a sofa. People aren't just hunched while using a tablet, they're often twisted like a pretzel. It sounds like a prescription for postural disaster, but there *is* one saving grace: The positions can be so awkward that users tend to grow uncomfortable much more quickly than they do while sitting at their desks. They're more likely to move, making the postural effects less damaging.

Even worse than being a desk jockey is being a couch potato. In many Western countries, watching TV is the most common activity, next to sleeping and working. TV viewing tends to be associated with many other unhealthy behaviors, such as snacking while viewing, poor sleep hygiene, and exposure to advertising for unhealthy foods. Too many people sit at work, sit in the car, and then sit at home—rinse and repeat, day after day.

Ancient DNA Meets Modern Life

How could something as basic to modern life as sitting cause so many health problems for so many people? The answer dates back 2.5 million to 3 million years, to the dawn of humankind. From then up until the agricultural revolution 10,000 years ago, human beings were opportunistic out of necessity, eating whatever they could get their hands on, as long as it was a wild plant or an animal. There wasn't much sitting around. Hunter-gatherers stayed in one place for a week or two, exhausting the available resources and then moving on. Over the course of a year, they might have exploited ten to thirty plant foods as staples and ten to fifteen species of animals or fish. When one kind of food went out of season or grew scarce, they found something else to eat.

Because of this lifestyle, the human body became very adept at conserving energy. When human ancestors ingested calories, their bodies clung to them, not knowing when or even if their next meal might come. The more calories their body stored, the longer they could go without food.

Fast-forward to modern times. While there are still hunter-gatherers roaming the Earth, such as the Bushmen of southern Africa and the Hadza of Tanzania, few humans now fit that description. Without discounting the harsh reality that a huge number of people go hungry today around the globe, for many people in the modern world, food now comes all too easily. There are more than 40,000 supermarkets and grocery stores and approximately 250,000 fast-food restaurants in the United States alone. If even the drive-through lane requires too much effort, delivery services will now bring your meal right to your doorstep. Food deliveries were a luxury before the coronavirus pandemic; now many people depend on them for their subsistence.

But the problem isn't just the ease of acquiring food; it's the makeup of that highly accessible food. To cite just one example, the average annual per capita consumption of sugar in the United States is 152 pounds, not to mention another 146 pounds of flour that converts directly to sugar. Sugar and flour are inexpensive, potent agents for storing fat, particularly when consumed to excess—and take it from me, 152 pounds is excessive. Sugar consumption changes your blood glucose levels and the hormone insulin in ways that increase hunger. So people keep eating the same foods that tend to promote fat storage.

These changes in food accessibility, procurement, and consumption have occurred at lightning speed relative to the snail-like pace of human evolution. We're still genetically programmed to hoard calories and store energy. Evolution thinks we're still scavenging for that next meal and at risk of starvation at any moment. So the calories pile up as unwanted pounds. Sitting is an activity that has less caloric burn and amplifies all of this.

Even more harmful than sitting for too long is sitting for too long in an awkward position. As people proceed through a typical day, they place themselves in awkward configurations and sometimes remain there for hours without reprieve. Instead of walking or running from point A to point B, they jam their bodies awkwardly into cars, trains, and planes. I'll use a friend of mine as an example. It all started innocuously enough, with a slight stiffening in his low back as he left Honolulu International Airport, where he'd landed for a getaway with his new girlfriend. It was his first trip to Hawaii. By the time he swiped his room key at the hotel, pain was building from his right gluteus down to his right foot. The pain and stiffness worsened over the next twenty-four hours. Barely able to hold on to his suitcase and hobbled by now-excruciating leg pain, my friend managed to make it back to the airport for a red-eye flight home. In the air, every turbulent bounce pushed him closer to passing out during what became the most miserable six hours of his life.

A day after my friend returned to the mainland, a chiropractor adjusted his spine and prescribed a pain med. When the pain gave way to numbness and he could no longer push off his right foot, my friend sought a second opinion from another spine doc. Pain is unpleasant, but what alarms medical professionals like me even more than pain is numbness and strength loss. Those are more serious symptoms and are potentially even permanent. This new spine doc quickly scheduled my friend for a consult with a neurosurgeon.

That next appointment made it clear that this was a medical emergency. "Your S1 nerve is dying," said the neurosurgeon, wide-eyed in the glow of the MRI he was analyzing. "We need to operate tomorrow. I'll get clearance from your insurer under 'loss of life, loss of limb.'" My friend's mind spun wildly. *Tomorrow? Loss of limb?* The neurosurgeon meant loss of function, not amputation, but still, my friend was floored. The disc between the two lowest vertebrae in his spine had ruptured on the plane, ejecting its jellylike filling. Complicating matters immeasurably, 80 percent of the disc material was now rubble heaped atop this pivotal nerve root, the S1, at the point where it tunneled from his pelvis into his right leg.

My friend limped out of the neurosurgeon's office, his shock compounded by how healthy and strong he'd felt right up to the injury. For four months straight, he'd charged through tough workouts with great results. Somehow everything changed on the airplane, which is a common venue for lumbar disc ruptures, as it turns out, in part because the ergonomics of the seats and the spaces between them are so bad. He was never my patient, but my guess is that four decades of hunching in front of a computer and careless lifting of everyday objects had gradually compromised his disc. Then it gave way.

The surgery went as well as it could have given the circumstances. Most of the nerve sensation in his right leg came back. Motor skill improvement would prove more elusive, returning only partially by the end of his rehabilitation. He was forbidden from lifting anything heavier than a coffee mug for a month; sitting, standing, bending, and rolling over in bed became elaborately choreographed acts. He caught a glimpse into the sense of claustrophobia, and panic that comes from the loss of movement—the movement many take for granted until they lose it.

My friend felt blindsided. But when I questioned him, his answers were riddled with obvious clues. He'd experienced twinges of pain in his lower back for several years, yet he chose to ignore them, wishfully thinking they'd disappear. He was working out during the weeks before the injury, which is great; everyone should exercise. But his strength coach was leading him through deadlifts and squats, as well as ballistic moves such as box jumps and squat jumps, which would be the recommended approach if he had been a high school football player. Instead, he was in his early fifties with a balky low back pinging his brain with red-alert signals. I wish I could have intervened back then, before it was too late.

DO THIS NOW: If you're tall, request an aisle seat or, better yet, an exit row or bulkhead seat on your next flight. The aisle seat will make it easier to stand up and walk a bit every hour or so. Being locked in an awkward position for hours is very stressful for your spine. The exit row seat will let you stretch your legs more easily. Even if you can't reserve one of those seats, flight attendants often will show mercy and seat tall passengers in exit rows.

3 SIXTEEN HEALTH LANDMINES RELATED TO BAD POSTURE

THE WORLD'S POPULATION is increasingly overweight, and the most frequently cited reasons are too many calories plus too little exercise. Indeed, those are both significant parts of the problem. But lack of dedicated exercise wouldn't be as big of an issue if people were more mobile in their everyday life. Unfortunately, instead of walking and moving around, they're sitting far too much. And I have noticed many orthopedic ailments as a result.

Most chronic pain and other modern-day maladies have a connection with excessive sitting and poor posture. The odds of contracting any of a variety of health problems and diseases such as heart disease, type 2 diabetes, stroke, degenerative disc disease, arthritis, sciatica, and osteoporosis all soar among those who sit too much. There tends to be something else at work, something specific to the act of prolonged sitting.

Let's tiptoe through these health landmines that I've observed in my orthopedic practice one by one to get a sense of what we're dealing with here.

Landmine No. 1: Weight Gain

Those who sit for much of the day burn fewer calories than active people, making them more prone to packing on pounds. Weight gain itself is a risk factor for many health problems, most obviously type 2 diabetes but also heart disease and cancer.

Weight gain isn't good for your posture, either. Having more weight around your waist will naturally change your center of mass and throw off your alignment. Some researchers have even suggested that being overweight reduces your foot's ability to feel the ground, therefore affecting your postural balance negatively. Being overweight also places a lot of pressure on bones and connective tissue, which strain to support a body much bigger than its skeletal system was designed to handle.

Landmine No. 2: Loss of Muscle and Strength

Humans naturally experience a decrease in skeletal muscle mass starting in their early thirties. This is medically known as sarcopenia. The older someone gets, the more pronounced this muscle-wasting process becomes. With decreased muscle mass comes a loss in strength and performance.

When people slouch in front of a screen for much of the day, muscles begin to atrophy from lack of use. Screen jockeys whose primary work activity is tapping keys can fight against this preprogrammed muscle loss by staying active. Lifting weights and engaging in other forms of resistance training are all beneficial in this regard. Muscle is the most metabolically active tissue in the human body, so even a body at rest burns calories to maintain itself. Remember when I said that standing all day doesn't turn you into a fat-burning machine? Well, carrying around muscle on your bones does. By not exercising to build muscle, you forfeit the chance to enlist muscle to help you in the fight against strength loss and poor posture.

Landmine No. 3: Weaker, More Brittle Bones

Physical activity puts muscles to work, and this work stimulates them to grow, but bones also require exercise to stay strong. Inactivity revs up a type of bone cell called an osteoclast that breaks down bone tissue. In contrast, physical activity reduces the rate of bone loss and helps conserve bone tissue. That explains why athletes tend to have higher bone mineral density and greater bone strength than other people.

In other words, it's "use it or lose it" when it comes to bone health. As with muscles, bones tend to weaken with age. It's already an uphill battle to keep them strong and healthy in later years. If you're inactive, the downhill slide will only accelerate, eventually leading to problems such as hip fractures and spinal compression fractures.

Landmine No. 4: Muscle Imbalances

Hunched posture and too much sitting weakens postural muscles, forcing the body to rely on the joints for support, which causes long-term damage (Figure 3.1). That's why it's important to focus on strengthening our postural muscles by maintaining good posture in sitting and standing. Doing so will place less stress on joints. This will lead to better movement and reduced pain.

With bad posture, some muscles become neurologically inhibited. As certain muscles cease doing their job correctly, others strain to compensate, causing other imbalances. Muscles that are chronically shortened or lengthened can't produce the force or sustain the endurance they normally would. Sitting incorrectly causes the body to grow accustomed to using muscles in a shortened range of motion. To understand the concept of range of motion, let your right arm hang down. Now bend your elbow to raise your forearm toward your shoulder, the same motion used to curl a dumbbell. Full range of motion should allow your fist to approach within inches of your shoulder. If your fist stops well short of your shoulder, your range of motion at the elbow joint is limited, not complete.

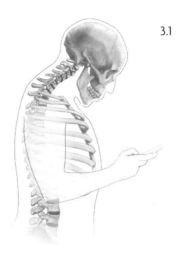

3.1

Phone use leading to head forward, hunched postures

Limited ranges of motion lead to the development of inefficient movement patterns that perpetuate stiffness and, in the long run, compromise your joints. If you sit all day with your thoracic spine slightly flexed, over time your body will become more efficient at being flexed. You'll get used to it, and problems won't immediately arrive when you're in that position. Instead, you'll turn your head while driving one day and awkwardly twist your neck in a bad way. And then you'll wonder: *How the hell did that happen?*

Landmine No. 5: Muscle Spasms

Muscle spasms occur when the body needs to protect something. This is seen in many cases of low back pain, the most common condition I see in the clinic. A spasm is a sudden involuntary tightening of the muscle, usually due to overuse or fatigue, electrolyte depletion, or a joint being stressed dangerously, like a dislocation or a fracture. When you're stuck in the same posture for a long period, your body adapts to the limited amount of movement. Try to move out of the posture suddenly, and you'll likely experience a protective muscle spasm. Conversely, if a muscle hasn't been used for a long time and is deconditioned, trying to use it more than it has been also may cause a spasm. This is the body's way of preventing you from injuring the muscle.

To avoid muscle spasms, train your muscles progressively, prevent dehydration, and move within safe ranges of motion that your body is familiar with.

DO THIS NOW: Favor free weights over machines at the gym. When you lift free weights, your stabilizer muscles need to pitch in to help your prime movers. Exercise machines remove the need for stabilizers to kick in because the machine offers support. If you use machines all the time, your main muscles will grow bigger and stronger, but your stabilizers won't keep up, potentially leading to spasms, pulls, and other injuries.

Landmine No. 6: Joint Stress

When postural muscles become weak, the body has no choice but to rely on joints for support, leading to long-term joint damage.

Every joint in the human body has an optimal position from which it operates at maximum efficiency. Consider the case of sprinter Usain Bolt. As he glides down the track, his movements are perfectly synchronized, to the point where sprinting at world-record speed looks effortless. That's because he is moving through his muscles, not through his joints. There is no wasted motion, no joint friction—just a human body moving exactly as it was designed to move. It's a beautiful sight to behold.

Chances are you'll never be the world's fastest human. However, like Bolt, you want your muscles, not your joints, to carry the load. The more you focus on using your muscles, the less reliant you'll become on your joints. This will lead to better movement throughout your body and reduced pain. Maintaining good posture is one of the best ways to help your body rely on its musculature while preserving your joints.

Landmine No. 7: Spine Pathologies

Even if a spine forms normally, changes can occur over time that begin compromising its structural integrity. When a person sits too long in an awkward position, pressure can steadily build on the spinal discs. When the normal spine curves start changing—most distressingly, when those trademark S curves flatten—the spine's structural elements are subjected to forces they weren't meant to handle. The spine becomes less adept at doing its many jobs.

A misaligned spine leads to disc compression and degeneration (Figure 3.2). A worsening of structural integrity usually includes those jelly-filled cushions flattening and bulging out to the sides. This disc material can begin pressing on the nerves running through the spine, leading to pain (e.g., sciatica) and even loss of function. Eventually, those discs can rupture, causing the disc material to push out into the spinal canal. This is exactly what happened to my friend on his flight to Hawaii. If we continue with the jelly doughnut analogy, it's like someone sat on the doughnut, causing the jelly to squirt out and make a mess. Only this mess can't be wiped up with a napkin. This debris in the spinal canal affects delicate nerves, and removing it surgically is a significant operation. Even if all goes well, the unavoidable bleeding and scar tissue from the surgery itself amounts to more foreign debris littering the spinal canal.

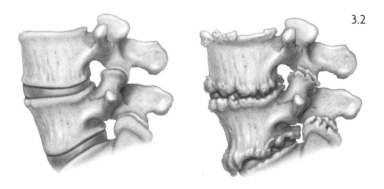

3.2

Damaged joints

To understand what's at stake when the spine is injured, you need to realize that any catastrophic break (like a terrible car accident or a traumatic fall) in the nerves traveling down the spinal curve renders the human body immobile below that point. The severity of the paralysis depends on the location of the spinal cord damage. A severe enough injury in the spine's cervical area can lead to quadriplegia, paralysis from at least the shoulders down. A severe enough injury occurring in the thoracic area can lead to paraplegia, paralysis of the legs and lower body.

Landmine No. 8: Pinched Nerves

Muscular imbalances, inefficient joints, and changes to the spine's natural S curves eventually can lead to pinched nerves. If you've experienced one, you know what I'm talking about; if you haven't, you'll know it when it happens. Not only can a pinched nerve be painful, but it can produce scary sensations such as tingling or numbness and even a loss of muscle function. Like bulging discs, a pinched nerve in the neck or shoulder can produce numbness that radiates down the arm.

I saw these particular symptoms a lot more early in my career before wireless headsets became commonplace. Back then, front desk workers and secretaries spent long stretches typing while on the phone, the handset jammed between their ear and shoulder. After many years spent working in that position, many of them developed pain and numbness radiating down their arms.

Break Glass When Needed!

QUICK-FIX LOW BACK STRETCH

After sitting at the computer for too long, do you find yourself experiencing pain or stiffness in the lower back? If so, tight hip flexors might be to blame. Located at the front of the hips, the hip flexors are the muscles that allow you to bend at the waist and lift your knees. These often become tight from sitting for long periods.

Try this simple stretch to help open up your body's front and reduce tension in the low back and hips:

1. Begin in a half-kneeling position, with one knee on the floor and the other leg bent 90 degrees in front of you (Figure 3.3).

2. Shift your hips forward until you feel a slight tension in the thigh of your kneeling leg.

3. Sweep both arms overhead to open up the front of the body further and lengthen the hip flexor (Figure 3.4).

4. Hold the stretch a few seconds for a total of five to six repetitions before switching sides. Try to move into the stretch a little deeper with each repetition.

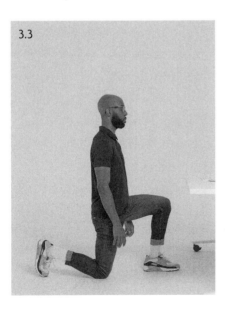
3.3

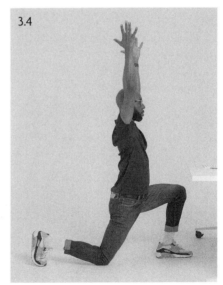
3.4

Landmine No. 9: Forward Head Posture

I see patients with neck pain all the time. And this is often due to forward head posture. The neck is extremely mobile; we're constantly flexing and rotating it. As with any part of the body subject to frequent use, the parts inside can wear out and deteriorate, especially when the spine and posture are misaligned. When we are trying to get the neck properly aligned, it's important not only to look at the neck but also to pay attention to what's going on in the shoulder girdle and the thoracic area.

Forward head posture (aka "tech neck") develops when the head leans forward to engage with cell phones, laptops, and other electronics. People in this situation tend to look forward and down simultaneously, causing the neck and thoracic spine to flex. The head tilts forward, out in front of the shoulder girdle's center, and the body's center of gravity shifts, causing the shoulders to round (Figures 3.5, 3.6). This forward head posture forces ligaments, not muscles, to begin supporting the head, which accounts for one-seventh of a human being's body weight. When the head moves too far forward, the neck muscles grow tired and irritated. No wonder so many people feel tightness in the back of their neck, in their upper back, and between their shoulder blades, and they experience so many headaches. More ominously, chronic forward head lean begins flattening the curve of the upper spine and neck.

The longer you sit in front of a computer or other device, the likelier you are to experience neck pain, and the worse it's likely to be. Five hours a day spent sitting at a desk seems to be a cutoff point, after which this sitting posture becomes a significant risk factor for neck pain. The screen is the crucial element here. An Iranian study found that staring at a computer screen for extended periods led to incorrect posture and neck pain. Yet when study subjects sat and looked at a point on a wall, rather than a computer screen, those neck issues didn't materialize.

Hunching while staring at a computer screen isn't the only cause of forward head posture. Even something as seemingly harmless as sleeping with pillows stacked too high may contribute. So can a lack of upper back strength.

Forward head posture isn't just a problem for office workers. Dentists, for example, also tend to develop forward head lean. Studies of dentists in Iran found that the percentage of them suffering from neck pain ranged from 28 to 61 percent. Neck pain can eventually turn into something chronic and even disabling.

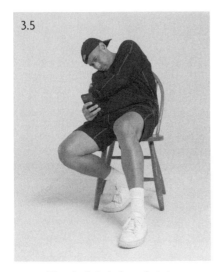

Slouched, imbalanced sitting

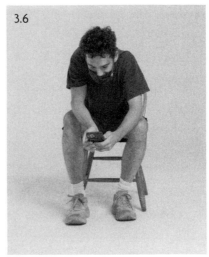

Rounded shoulders through phone use

Landmine No. 10: Movement Compensation

I want you to try something at home. Open a closet or cupboard and reach for the highest item in there. Now grab your phone and look down at it as you reach for the same thing. Are you able to reach as far? Did it get a bit harder? That's because while looking at your phone, you changed your posture. How? Your neck flexed and your middle back and shoulders rounded, biomechanically reducing your capacity to reach overhead. What does that say about posture? It influences how you move your shoulders. And with poor posture comes compensation with your movement. Let's explore this with the shoulder.

When you think about shoulder pain and injuries, what likely comes to mind first are those related to sports and occupations. The gym-goer loading too much weight onto the barbell for a shoulder press. Or the delivery driver reaching up awkwardly for a heavy package. But the shoulder can be stressed *anywhere*. Think about what happens when a mom reaches for something while her kid tugs on her other arm. Before I even start treating the shoulder girdle, I assess the whole body, starting with posture.

Shoulder injuries are difficult to fix and rehabilitate, because like the spine, the shoulder must be simultaneously flexible in several planes of movement and highly stable, yet capable of handling heavy loads. Its ball-and-socket joint has a supporting cast of bones, muscles, and ligaments inside and outside of the joint capsule. There's a lot that can go wrong, from soft tissue injuries and bone disease to joint impairment and instability. But often times the shoulder can be injured because of excessive load due to compensation of other muscles working more than they should.

Acute injuries like those befalling the delivery driver happen every day. Yet shoulder pain and dysfunction also arise slowly from poor posture, and movement compensation. This gradual degeneration and compensation leads directly to acute injuries. For example, a rounded mid back can increase your risk for a tendon tear at the shoulder.

When it comes to shoulder pain, rib cage alignment is an overlooked cause. If your rib cage position is off, it will change the position of your shoulder blades and decrease the space between the ball-and-socket joint and the uppermost shoulder bone. This may lead to impingement and other shoulder dysfunctions. Like the pelvis, the rib cage can tilt forward or backward. The vertebrae that attach to the ribs are the thoracic vertebrae, so it's no wonder that people with an unusual positioning of their rib cage also tend to have a stiff thoracic spine.

Landmine No. 11: Immobility and Energy Drain

The hip flexors, the set of muscles near the top of the thighs, tighten when you sit at a desk for long stretches. Once you get up and start walking with tight hip flexors, you can't reach full stride. Your body needs to compensate by rotating the torso enough to achieve a normal walking stride.

Mobility tends to feed on itself. If you're mobile all day, it's easier to keep being mobile, whereas if you're sedentary all day, being mobile becomes a bigger deal than it needs to be. This can then have a negative effect on your energy.

DO THIS NOW: Start following a daily walking regimen. I'm a big believer in taking three fifteen-minute walks a day: morning, afternoon, and evening. During the workday, take your meetings while walking. These walks will clear your head, stimulate creativity, lubricate your joints, burn a few calories, and keep your hip flexors more limber. Along with drinking water, taking regular walks might be the best thing you can do for your body. It's a game changer!

Excessive sitting and bad posture can both sap your energy. Think of it this way: If I forced you to go through the day wearing handcuffs, you would expend a ton of energy trying to navigate your daily activities. Everything would take extra effort. Likewise, with bad posture, the body has to work harder to overcome inefficiencies.

Bad posture is like those handcuffs positioned all around your body. You expend a lot of energy trying to move with them and feel exhausted by day's end.

Landmine No. 12: Moods and Self-Esteem

Slouching affects people emotionally as well as physically. According to an article in the *New York Times*, studies have shown that people with clinical depression tend to adopt a hunched posture. Not only can a hunched posture reflect depression, but it also can make it harder for someone who is depressed to begin feeling better. Also, scientists at the University of Amsterdam in the Netherlands found that study subjects with a slouched posture had a more difficult time pulling themselves out of a bad mood than subjects who sat up straight.

When people see someone with good posture, they also see confidence, command, and other positive attributes. When people see someone hunch, they perceive a lack of confidence, sadness, and fear. This becomes a feedback loop: When someone's posture is good, people respond positively; when it's bad, they respond negatively, all of which reinforces the person's posture. Little wonder, then, that bad posture and low self-esteem are highly correlated.

I've noticed in my physical therapy practice at Myodetox how past experiences can influence a person's posture in ways they may not even realize. Long after troubling events such as abuse and physical pain from accidents have passed, someone can still hold on to a hunched and guarded posture as a protective mechanism.

I find that there is both physical and mental strife in nearly every patient I see with chronic pain issues. I tend to focus on posture and biomechanics before I start looking at their mind and their emotions. Like most people in my profession, I was trained to be *physical* in my physical therapy. Often, though, I realize other factors are at play: depression, anxiety, childhood trauma, relationship issues, or some other stress. Eight out of ten U.S. adults say they experience stress in their daily lives. I'm sure that percentage has risen during these troubling times.

I remember one client who came to see me at my clinic in Toronto with neck pain. "It's killing me," she said.

At the end of our first session, I said, "Your neck is stiff, but the good news is there doesn't seem to be anything structurally wrong." We completed two or three more sessions, which did nothing to change my initial diagnosis. Her neck seemed okay.

Midway through our fourth session, out of nowhere, she exclaimed, "My husband's cheating on me!" She began sobbing.

I have reasonably good people skills, so I consoled her as best I could, well aware that I'm neither a psychologist nor a relationship expert. At that moment, I just tried to be an empathetic human being. I came to realize that, while her neck *was* stiff—probably from the jaw-clenching stress of her situation—what she needed was someone to talk to, a person slightly removed from her personal life, not a close friend or family member. By the end of that fourth session, her pain was gone, and not because of any treatment I provided. I just listened.

Landmine No. 13: Disrupted Sleep

Everything I've discussed here, from aches and pains to pinched nerves, can keep you awake at night. How can you sleep soundly if your body can't relax?

An analysis of many related studies published in the *International Journal of Behavioral Medicine* found that prolonged sedentary behavior elevates the risk of insomnia. Poor sleep can weaken the immune system and lead to serious medical conditions, such as heart disease, hypertension, and type 2 diabetes. Sleep deprivation of just two hours a night doubles your obesity risk. Sleep disruption also leads to increased hunger and decreased satiety, because it prompts changes in the appetite-regulating chemical messengers ghrelin and leptin.

More immediately, poor sleep can interfere with everything from work productivity to quality of life, including your sex life. "After a night of tossing and turning, you may feel more irritable, short-tempered, and vulnerable to stress the next day," says James Yoon, ND, a naturopathic physician. Everyone wants to rise from bed and start their day feeling energized and refreshed, ready to take on life's challenges. If you're already yawning by breakfast, though, and you need three cups of coffee just to get going, you won't be at your best as the day unwinds. The resulting subpar performance could be rooted in poor sleep caused, or worsened, by poor posture.

Landmine No. 14: Lack of Motivation

"The zone" refers to that state of being during competition where the body, mind, and emotions are so perfectly in sync that everything falls into place, seemingly with ease. Athletes talk about the game slowing down, almost to slow motion, in this state. Others say that when they are in the zone, the basket or goal looks twice as big as it actually is, making them feel like they can't miss. Those who routinely enter the zone are labeled clutch performers, in contrast to those who are labeled chokers because they're stressed rather than relaxed in crunch time.

It's not only possible but also desirable to be in the zone at work, too. Instead of crawling, time seems to fly by. Ideas come easily. You feel highly motivated, even if you can't articulate why. Whatever you do for a living, your work product is exceptional in this state, and you receive all the kudos and rewards that come with being regarded as a peak performer.

People in the zone aren't hunched over at their computer; they're sitting up straight, alert, locked in. And because they sit in this fashion, they aren't dogged by the many health problems I've outlined.

You can't end up in the zone at work, though, if you're preoccupied by pain. The greater the pain, the greater the distraction. Anyone who has tried to focus on something else while in tremendous pain knows how challenging it is. Chronic pain sufferers deal with a phenomenon called attentional bias, which refers to unconsciously searching the surrounding environment for elements that will either alleviate (palliatives) or exacerbate (threats) the pain. This preoccupation with pain makes it very difficult for the sufferer to focus on even the most mundane tasks.

Landmine No. 15: Poor Balance

At Myodetox, a large portion of our patients are older. And falls are the leading cause of injuries among the elderly. Because the elderly often have fragile skeletons, a fall that a younger person could shake off with ease—or that would never happen in the first place—can harm an older person. Falls also can leave them in the terrifying predicament of being unable to get back up or call for help.

Some older individuals are more prone to falling than others. One problem is that the elderly often lose their ability to move laterally quickly or while maintaining their balance. They don't operate well in the frontal plane. Life, of course, happens in multiple planes, so when they do need to move laterally—say, they get bumped or they trip—their body can't adjust quickly enough, and they fall. The curves of the spine play a significant role in this phenomenon. In studies of those sixty-five years of age and older, the more distorted the curve of someone's spine, the more likely they are to fall. As I've discussed, a compromised spinal curve comes from years, even decades, of bad posture. Working on your posture now lessens the chances of broken bones later in life.

Landmine No. 16: Impaired Breathing

A slouched or collapsed sitting posture compresses the lungs and impedes the diaphragm, the large, dome-shaped muscle that forms the floor of the rib cage and powers breathing. As a result, hunching makes breathing more shallow and less efficient. Even if you don't notice it, shallow breathing is bad for your heart and brain, which needs a steady flow of oxygen for survival, let alone peak performance. Even worse for your lungs is curling up in a C position with your laptop for long stretches.

In contrast, when you sit or stand up straight, the lungs and diaphragm have the breathing room to do what they were designed to do. The resulting deep, sustained breaths support and nourish the entire body.

Choosing a Different Path

Poor posture and lousy mobility become a self-fulfilling prophecy for millions of people. They become less active, grow depressed, get sick, and start to hunch, making them more depressed. But there's a much rosier future ahead if you follow a different path, one where you take better care of yourself. A Myodetox investor named David offers Exhibit A. David hadn't reached rock bottom; still, in middle age, he'd become resigned to a life of disability and lingering health problems, rooted in a car accident that occurred in his teens when he broke both ankles. The right one was particularly damaged and needed to be fused, keeping the ankle intact but causing him to limp. David's body naturally compensated for the injury, leading to problems with his knees and lower back. In adulthood, this mega-successful entrepreneur hated having to drag around his leg.

David and I met face-to-face in Vancouver when I was looking for investors in Myodetox. I ended up treating him every day for a week. I couldn't un-fuse his ankle, but I found that tightness in his big toe, of all things, was making matters worse. That's where I focused my treatment. David's wife was on hand, too, and after a few days, she said, "Wow, David, you're walking so much better now!" You could just see his spirit lift as his mobility improved.

David's only regret is that he didn't prioritize his health earlier. Part of the disconnect is cultural. When David was a young man, "wealth" was measured by the size of someone's bank account. And he went on to make a fortune establishing a near-monopoly in restaurant franchises in Hawaii. As is true of many men of his generation, though, his body was just along for the ride until it finally gave way. Today, most of us realize that self-actualization has little to do with numbers on a bank statement and everything to do with how you feel and your quality of life.

So in the race to become healthier, people have turned to fitness. Gyms and boutique fitness studios are now fixtures in strip malls. These facilities are doing their best based on the information they have available, but many still equate "health" with "moving a lot of plates," "going for the burn," or six-pack abs. They market a "push, push, push" narrative, and while this encourages activity, which is a good thing, employees at some of these trendy fitness chains don't always understand the body. Specifically, they have a blind spot when it comes to recovery and proper spinal hygiene routines. Unwittingly, sometimes they *break* the body they seek to improve, replacing motivation with disillusionment. If you think it's hard to get someone into fitness once, try doing it twice, after an injury.

Health is so much more than "push, push, push." At Myodetox, we fix. We rebuild. We empower people to improve and extend their life. My message boils down to "Push, take a break, push, sleep, push harder and smarter." I don't promise a six-pack, but I'm offering you something more valuable: more time to do the things you love, as well as the ability to do them pain-free. The more conscientiously you futureproof your body, the longer you'll move well, and the longer you'll live. Life is awesome. It should last as long as humanly possible.

But along with longevity, it's about quality of life. I want you to live to eighty, ninety, a hundred years old, but I don't want you to live that long sitting in a wheelchair or shuffling from the bed to the bathroom and back. I want you to enjoy and celebrate your longevity. I want you to be fulfilled and self-actualized. Most of all, I want you to be pain-free.

4 | MOVEMENT IS LIFE

THE FITNESS INDUSTRY was built on changing the human body's shape through burning fat and building muscle. We've all seen before-and-after transformation photos in magazine articles and ads, featuring moment-in-time views of the same person, heavier juxtaposed with thinner/healthier/happier. But until this decade, what was an afterthought was how the body moves when it's not lifting weights or running.

We move spontaneously and fluidly all the time when we're very young, but as we mature, efficiency and technology take over. (By the way, this transition to tech is now starting as early as kindergarten in some cases.) We buy a car, so there's no longer any compelling need to walk. We get a job, but instead of the manual labor of a teen's summer job, we're planted behind a desk. "*Climbing* the corporate ladder" is an often used expression, ironic, given that there's barely any physical activity happening in sedentary office jobs.

Even when most people work out, they tap only a fraction of their body's potential. There's nothing wrong with doing leg extensions or a simple hamstring stretch, but life's challenges seldom unfold in a single plane of movement. Think of what muscles are asked to do in obstacle races like Spartan or Tough Mudder: surmounting wooden barriers and crawling through mud under barbed wire require more varied training than just barbell squats, biceps curls, or stretching. In life, you need to be ready for whatever comes your way.

DO THIS NOW: Use a basket instead of a shopping cart. The cart is designed to make life easier, but it does next to nothing to improve mobility. However, if you're carrying around a basket, it becomes a loaded carry like a farmer's walk. Better still, the load is being held in one hand, forcing your core to brace to stabilize your torso.

Earlier I mentioned Bruce Lee. I admired Bruce's strength, flexibility, combat skills, coordination, discipline, dedication, and charisma, all of which were extraordinary. But if there was one thing I admired about Lee above all else, it was how fluidly he moved. He made the impossible look effortless. This statement may reflect my bias as a physical therapist, but I view Bruce Lee as an icon of movement first and foremost.

On-screen, Bruce's muscular and ripped physique was the center of attention. But to achieve his extreme mobility, his muscles had to work in perfect harmony with the other structures in his body, starting with his joints. The body contains more than 250 such "hinges." Joints contain a viscous fluid designed to reduce friction by keeping hard, bony surfaces and cartilage from grinding against one another, much as the engine oil in a car's crankcase keeps heat and friction from burning up the engine. This joint fluid does more than lubricate, though. It's like a delivery truck that helps transport nutrients into joints and then loads up waste products and takes them away.

Rheumatoid arthritis, a disease in which the body's immune system attacks those joints, leaving them swollen and inflamed, illustrates the delicacy and vulnerability of the joints in the human body. You can see joint damage in the gnarled hands of someone who has been dealing with the disease for many years. Sadly, the disease is as painful as it looks. That's one source of joint pain, and it's the one physical therapists like me can't do much about, unfortunately. Patients rely on powerful immune-suppressing drugs that have a lot of nasty side effects.

Another source of pain at the joint region is bone fractures and tears to ligaments and cartilage. Any sports fan knows what joint injuries mean for athletes. An injury to the anterior cruciate ligament, or ACL, strikes fear in the hearts of players and fans alike. Those three letters signify a severe knee injury involving long rehabilitation, with no guarantee that the athlete will recapture their past form with a reconstructed knee. Injuries like that, I can help with—both prevention and recovery. But in sports there's no way to entirely avoid them. Take football, for example: When a running back hits the line and 300-pounders start landing on him awkwardly, bad things can happen.

Prepare Your Mind to Heal Your Body

A number of you reading this book will be doing so because you're coming back from an injury, perhaps more than one injury. And in that case, while you'll still be futureproofing your body, you'll also be rehabbing injuries that have already occurred. Obviously, there are medical and physical therapy challenges involved in doing both at once. Hopefully this book can help augment whatever you're doing. Most doctors would say that the routines I offer will be beneficial for somebody coming back from an injury.

One thing I don't think receives enough attention is the *psychology* of rehabbing an injury. Injuries are shocking events for most people. If you've been through one, you know what I'm talking about. They come out of left field and shake you to your foundation because they rob you of things you've taken for granted your whole life, like movement.

But it's important to do what you need to do to get back to where you were. Most people experience injuries, so you're certainly not alone in having to deal with one. The longer you wait, the harder it is to get back to where you were before. It's better to bite the bullet, do what you need to do, and develop the mind-set that what has occurred is merely an interruption on a journey. Think of it as turbulence on a flight. It seems unsettling at the time, but it doesn't have to deter you from reaching your destination.

When you are trying to avoid joint diseases, sports injuries, and excessive wear and tear, it helps to start early. I'll give you an example. A patient I'll call Julia came to me with back pain when she was only twenty-one years old. From the moment we met, she seemed defeated. She explained that pain had shot down her right leg for the previous five years whenever she tried to run. I learned that her chiropractor had told her at age sixteen that her joints weren't made for running. He actually told her point-blank that she should never run.

Negative feedback from such a trusted source had instilled in her an intense fear of movement. Eventually the feedback became a self-fulfilling prophecy. It's tough to deal with mobility issues early because empathy and understanding are in short supply. You're young; barring any obvious, visible disability, people think a twenty-one-year-old shouldn't have those sorts of issues.

It took intensive work over three to six months, but I was able to get Julia pain-free and running again with no problems.

Like Julia before she came to see me, most people use a fraction of their joint capacity in their daily life because of their limited mobility. They sit, stand up, lie down, get behind the wheel of a car, and so on. Very little of that activity puts their body through the various ranges of motion it's capable of.

Good mobility depends on having healthy joints. We tend to focus on using our muscles to perform exercise, whether lifting a weighted object or running on the pavement. Most of us don't think twice about our joints—until they begin hurting. If you're pounding the pavement on daily runs, your ankles and knee joints eventually start to ache. If you bench-press three times a week, your shoulder joints soon grow cranky. I'm proposing that you focus on your joints preemptively and for their own sake, before they become painful. The way to save your joints is to clean up your movement patterns, and the way to clean up your movement patterns is to use my posture hygiene plan.

A Mysterious Substance Holds the Key

There's actually an even more overlooked body component than joints—one that's pivotal to movement: fascia. I came upon it in 2010 while working as a teacher's assistant under Thomas Myers, a legend in the field of manual therapy who became one of my mentors. He advocated a holistic, integrative approach to treatment, which at the time was a maverick philosophy rather than a cliché. Working with Myers made me view the human body as a fully integrated system, and when I did, things suddenly began making sense.

The traditional rehab model took therapists through a series of if/then scenarios:

▶ If a muscle is weak, then strengthen it.

▶ If a muscle is tight, then stretch it.

Sometimes that worked. But what if it didn't? What if the muscle wasn't weak or tight, yet the person still couldn't move properly? I wanted to be able to do more than plead ignorance and dispatch patients unhealed.

Myers had a particular fascination, bordering on obsession, with what at the time seemed like an innocuous element in the human body. In the early days of medical research when scientists began dissecting bodies, they encountered a white substance that appeared to serve no apparent purpose. Everyone thought it was useless filler—human packing material that just took up space. This substance turned out to be vital to how our body moves (Figure 4.1).

Fascia is actually a network of microscopically thin membranes, and it's much more than filler. It's the "stitching" that holds together the human body's skin, muscle, and bone. It functions like the white transparent membrane you cut through on a chicken breast, or that white gooey stuff between the skin and the pulp you encounter when peeling an orange. Without that webbing, the fruit would fall apart. Likewise, without fascia, the human body would fold like a rag doll.

4.1

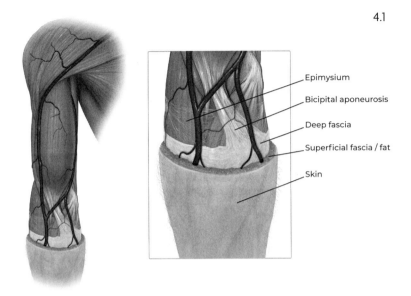

Epimysium

Bicipital aponeurosis

Deep fascia

Superficial fascia / fat

Skin

Fascia at the muscle level. "Human packaging material"

Usually, muscles move smoothly against other muscles because they're all surrounded by fascia. In addition to sheathing the outside of muscles, fascia surrounds the constituent parts, including the individual fibers bundled into muscles and the bundles themselves. Where muscle ends, fascia merges to form tendons, which connect muscle to bone.

Like a machine suffering the ill effects of friction, the microscopic boundaries between these elements can become less fluid, and hence less effective. When a related pair of muscles such as the biceps and the triceps—which alternately contract and lengthen in opposition to each other—falls out of balance, the fascia separating them can begin to harden. Eventually it can fuse in places, forming painful adhesions called trigger points. As the unbalanced musculature tries to adapt, fascia is further disrupted, producing more adhesions.

Fascia is also compromised by scar tissue, which forms any time muscles tear. It doesn't have to be something as catastrophic as a torn biceps, either; even micro-tears of the sort caused by repetitive lifting heal with scar tissue. Unfortunately, the scar tissue isn't as flexible or robust as the healthy tissue it replaces.

Once fascia is compromised, your body's ability to generate speed and power nose-dives. Your athletic performance will suffer as a result.

Myers has devoted much of his professional life to exploring the purpose and function of fascia. Under his tutelage, I became obsessed with it, too. Myers also opened my eyes to new areas of treatment. Let's say someone comes into one of our clinics because they can't go deep enough when they squat. They can't achieve ankle dorsiflexion, which is the backward bending of the foot. Is it because their nervous system won't allow them out of fear or past injury? Is it because they don't have the strength to go down? Is it because their calves are tight? Or is it because their fascial system lacks integrity? There are all sorts of potential reasons why someone can't go into a deep squat, and damaged fascia is one possible cause that not many physical therapists stop to consider.

One of my physical therapy goals is to improve the health of the myofascial system, the combined system of muscle and fascia. Applying intentional specific mechanical stress to this system through manual therapy or movement realigns and hydrates the fascia, allowing the layers to slide freely again. A massage might help to some degree, but usually, that's not enough. Many massage therapists press downward but don't know how to reach the layers they need to create the desired gliding effect. A therapist doesn't need to be heavy-handed when doing fascial work. It's more important to be precise. The questions I consider when I work on a patient are: *Should I push up or down the quads? Should I release this muscle or strengthen it? How will this affect their movement patterns?*

Mobility Training: Preventative Maintenance for Your Body

Now that you understand muscles, joints, and fascia, we can talk about mobility training. I mentioned earlier that fascia exists to balance mobility and muscular strength. Mobility by itself won't generate sufficient power for certain pursuits. For example, if you want to jump higher, squatting deeper isn't going to cut it. However, if all you do is squat heavy by adding more and more weight with limited mobility (e.g., squatting heavy and going down to barstool height), you won't be able to jump higher. You can lift heavy, but the force generated is limited and won't translate to a better jump. Therefore, finding the middle ground is key. This is where mobility training comes into play.

People have been lifting weights, doing calisthenics, and stretching since well back into the twentieth century, but widespread mobility training is a recent phenomenon. One fitness trend that has raised its profile is the popularity of CrossFit. Millions of people have taken up this sport, and many quickly realize they must improve their mobility if they want to train this way without getting injured.

Powerful forces conspire to keep us from being as mobile as we should. Sitting in front of a computer, in an airplane seat, behind a steering wheel—none of these are natural positions for the human body. Beyond external factors, aging itself works against good mobility, causing tissues to become less elastic and bones to grow more brittle. Chronic diseases such as type 2 diabetes and arthritis—any chronic pain syndrome, really—limit further mobility. Parkinson's disease and multiple sclerosis can make it difficult simply to walk. Of course, I'm not saying my posture regimen will offset those sorts of life-altering health conditions. Life poses particular challenges you must deal with as best you can. But for most people, these mobility exercises will be beneficial.

DO THIS NOW: Find ways to be more mobile in your everyday life. Running up three flights of stairs instead of stepping onto an escalator is a cliché, but choices like that can be very helpful. Opting into activity like that is a chance to strengthen your heart and muscles. Researchers at McMaster University in Canada are hardly the only ones to find that climbing stairs three times a week improves cardio-respiratory fitness. It's also a great leg and glute workout.

Another example is parking near the back of the lot and walking to the store, instead of sitting there for ten minutes with your car idling in hopes of grabbing the first spot. Bonus: No one's ever going to ding your car door if you're parked off by yourself.

Mobility training is ongoing preventive maintenance for the body, which is why it's essential to do it every day, even several times a day. It's about learning how to move freely and efficiently, and who doesn't want that? Mobility training reduces injury risk, improves joint health, and reduces joint pain. It mimics what you do in your everyday life, unlike bench pressing and touching your toes. Any time you move, any time you reach for or grab something, any time something unexpected comes your way, your body must be able to move in response. Which is to say, these exercises you're doing here will hold you in good stead in life.

Mobility is also essential because it's the thing that helps you promote stability and control of the muscles surrounding each of your joints. Mobility drills promote balance and the sense of where your body is in space. This sense will grow increasingly important as you age and become more prone to falls. Being able to maintain balance is essential for long-term quality of life and good health.

Mobility training also will help with your stability, which is related to but different from balance. Stability refers to the ability to stay grounded and strong while you perform a movement, whether that's lifting a package on your doorstep or hoisting a loaded barbell. For example, if you descend into a squat with a loaded barbell on your back, and your torso and extremities are shaking the entire time, you may be balanced, but you're not very stable. The drills I'll shortly be unveiling will help build stability so that when you do something like a barbell bench press or a squat, your movements will be safer and produce better results.

These movements might feel new and awkward. If you see somebody doing them in the gym, the shifting positions might look a little bit strange. That doesn't mean they aren't highly effective.

I like mobility training because it tends to recruit numerous sets of joints. Again, this reflects the demands and realities of everyday life. If you're doing a barbell curl, only one set of joints, your elbows, should be moving. But in life, we seldom use just one set of joints at a time. We almost always use multiple sets of joints simultaneously and in a coordinated fashion, which is why these exercises mimic that tendency.

Similar but Different: Mobility Versus Flexibility

Many people equate flexibility with mobility, but they're different. Flexibility refers to the range of movement available through a joint, whereas mobility refers to the extent to which your joints and muscles can move. Mobility involves strength, coordination, and body awareness. I'll give you a simple example. Lie on your back and bring your right knee toward your chest, using your hands to help. Note how close your knee comes to your chest. Now, without using your hands, again bring your right knee to your chest. I'm guessing you can't go as far without your hands helping you! This is an example of a joint having decent flexibility but limited mobility. I've designed my exercise program to improve flexibility *and* mobility.

You may have heard the term "static stretching," which is a type of stretching that promotes flexibility. An example would be reaching down and trying to touch your toes, and holding for thirty seconds. Without stretching, your muscles shorten and become tight and more injury prone. Dynamic stretching is also essential, and that's entering the realm of mobility. Dynamic stretching involves quicker holds (think 1 to 3 seconds). Dynamic equals mobility; static equals flexibility. One key difference between static and dynamic stretching is where you place them relative to your resistance training. As mentioned, dynamic stretching can be a very effective warm-up because it makes your tissues more elastic, raises your core temperature, and gets fluid moving in and out of your joints. Muscles and tendons possess a property called viscoelasticity, whereby they behave differently at different temperatures. Think of a piece of taffy: When it's cold, it's brittle, and if you tap it on the floor, it'll shatter. Warm it up, though, and it stretches rather than breaking or tearing. Your muscles are the same way: When they're warmer, they're less likely to get injured.

Dynamic stretches usually lead to an elevation in heart rate; static stretching does not. Static stretching doesn't get you moving. It doesn't make for a good warm-up activity because it doesn't elevate your body's heart rate or core temperature. There's also been some research suggesting that static stretches can actually *decrease* your ability to produce force in your workouts. So, for example, if you do a static stretch of the quadriceps before doing squats, your strength and power might diminish during the movement simply because you have stretched your quads beforehand. Again, this is a great reason to save a static quad stretch for *after* the workout, once your core temperature is elevated and your tissues are elastic. That's a much better time to be focused on lengthening tissues.

Static stretching should be gentle, not aggressive or ballistic. I see a lot of people forcing the action instead of coaxing their muscles into these positions. The classic example is somebody reaching down to try and touch their toes, only to have their hands stop at their shins. Frustrated, they bounce up and down to try and force progress. That's not the way to extend your range of motion. The only thing bouncing does is increase the risk of an injury—which defeats the purpose of the activity, since part of the reason for stretching is injury prevention.

DO THIS NOW: Stretch between your sets at the gym. Except when circuit training, you should have anywhere from thirty seconds to several minutes of downtime between sets. Use that time to perform static stretches. First, it's a highly efficient use of your valuable time. You're in the gym during those breaks between sets anyway, so use it. Second, as you proceed through a workout, your body temperature rises. Your tissues grow more elastic. So it's a great time to stretch.

I recommend stretching a body part other than the one being trained at that moment. If you're doing bench presses, I wouldn't recommend stretching your chest in between those sets because some research shows that stretching before a lift will decrease your force output. If you're doing a chest exercise, stretch your back in between those sets, then vice versa.

Genetics plays a role in how flexible you are. If you see an elite gymnast doing the splits on the balance beam, you may think to yourself, *I could never, ever do that,* which is quite possibly true. There are genetic freaks when it comes to flexibility, and top gymnasts are among them. But the point is that no matter our genetic limitations, we can all improve our flexibility. Your goal shouldn't be becoming as flexible as an Olympic athlete. It should be to become more flexible than before you started stretching or doing a program like mine.

The Big Consequences of Small Adjustments

And while we're speaking of elite athletes, several years ago, someone reached out to me and wrote, "Yohan Blake wants to see you."

I asked myself, *Why do I recognize this name?* So I searched "Yohan Blake" online. *Oh, man, I remember him!* He'd been a top sprinter, but I noticed he hadn't competed in three out of the past four years. I was busy at the time and didn't get the chance to respond immediately to the request to see him.

At some point, I said in passing to another Myodetox therapist: "Hey, you're into track and field, right? Have you heard of a guy named Yohan Blake? I'm supposed to link up with him, but he hasn't competed in nearly four years and I have so much going on."

The therapist looked at me, nearly cross-eyed in disbelief. "You're joking, right?" he asked. "Yohan Blake competes every year, Vinh, but he also competes every four years in the *Olympics*. He's one of the fastest men alive, and he's competing for Brazil in the upcoming Summer Games."

Feeling silly and pretty ignorant (it turns out, actually, that Yohan is the second fastest 100-meter man ever, behind Usain Bolt), I connected with Yohan's coach, Jae—the person who'd reached out. He offered to fly me to work with Yohan, who was then dealing with some nagging hamstring issues—obviously, a big deal for a sprinter training for the Olympics.

"I'll be honest," I said. "I don't want to mess with Yohan's mechanics a month before the Olympics. It's too close. If I'm going to work with him, it should be during his off-season."

Eventually, after the Olympics, I did go to Jamaica to work with Yohan. At the first training session I attended, he was doing various drills such as split jumps and sprints. His right foot kept angling outward, frustrating his coach to no end. Any issues with mechanics can be a fatal flaw for an elite sprinter.

After watching Yohan go back and forth with his coach for a while, I had to speak up. "Can I look at your foot for a second, Yohan?" I asked him to raise his toes, only some of which even came up. So I took him aside and did some quick physical therapy on his foot, digging into several small muscles that seemed to be locked up. After ten minutes of this, he tried the drills and sprints again. This time his right foot worked perfectly.

I share this story to illustrate the outsize importance of small things, like how your big toe functions relative to the rest of your body. I'm guessing that you've never paid a moment's attention to how your big toe works in your daily life. There are six hundred or so muscles in the human body. Many are so small and obscure that you may never have heard of them before or felt them being used until an unfamiliar activity makes them hurt. But many of those muscles that you didn't even know existed are very important, something you don't appreciate until something goes wrong.

The muscles of your big toe are a good example. If they get tight, if you don't stretch them, they can lead to all sorts of problems like the ones that were plaguing Yohan Blake.

I specialize in zeroing in on parts of the human body that many people don't even think about. If all you needed to do to stay functional and in peak shape was to exercise and stretch your quads, lats, and chest, you wouldn't need me. Anyone can do those sorts of things on their own. Yet the body is so much more complex than that. So as you progress through my posture hygiene routine, you'll discover that some of these exercises focus on areas you didn't think about before, like your toes; or the smaller muscles of the hips and glutes; or the intricate muscles in the middle of your back next to the lats.

5 | UNDERSTANDING WHERE YOU STAND

THE POSTURE AND MOBILITY PLAN outlined in this book should benefit *everyone*—certainly it shouldn't harm anyone. That said, everyone who follows the program will begin from a unique place. Often that starting point includes limitations that must be accounted for and worked around where necessary.

I'll share an example of what I mean. Early in my career, before the founding of Myodetox, I would travel from Toronto to Los Angeles to treat people I'd connected with on social media platforms. These physical therapy "barnstorming tours" grew out of a desire to help people who needed it while spreading the word about my approach. I didn't charge anyone anything. I just did it to meet people, hone my craft, and spread the word.

Before one trip, a guy who formerly served in the army hit me up on Instagram. His name was Grant. "Listen," he wrote, "my shoulder is bothering me, and I'm scheduled for surgery next week. I don't want to go through with it, but I don't know what else I can do. Can you help me?"

"I'll be honest, I don't know if I can help you," I wrote back. "But I'm willing to try, and it so happens I'm going to be in L.A. next week. Let's meet up."

I ended up meeting Grant in the Venice Beach area, where I'd set up a treatment table outside a friend's place where I was staying. As I said, I was doing this on the fly, and I didn't have an actual office space for seeing patients.

Before undertaking any therapy, I always seek a good understanding of what's going on. "I used to be able to do so many push-ups and pull-ups," he said, referencing bodyweight exercises favored in physical education classes and the military. "But then my right shoulder started hurting me. It's gotten to the point where I can't do a single pull-up now. The doctor who scheduled me for surgery says I have a rotator cuff problem."

Near where I'd set up my treatment table stood a small cluster of trees. Their leaves rustled in the ocean breeze.

"See that tree over there?" I asked. "I want you to try doing a pull-up on one of the lower branches. Just one rep."

"Sure," he said uneasily, "I'll give it a try."

He walked over to the tree and jumped to grab the lowest branch using an overhand grip. Grant hung for a moment before trying to pull himself up, only to grunt as the shoulder pain kicked in. After a pause, he tried to pull himself up again and then let go, landing back on the ground. He turned to me and shook his head in frustration.

I went over to him and began prodding around his right shoulder, zeroing in on the infraspinatus and supraspinatus, two small but important muscles that would be involved in what he'd just attempted to do. I could tell by his failed attempt that they were the likely culprits. Sure enough, they were tight as hell, practically locked up. I could feel trigger points as my fingertips dug into his flesh.

I had him do a few exercises to loosen those tight muscles, which he dutifully performed. After twenty minutes, I had him move his right shoulder through various ranges of motion.

"How does that feel?" I asked.

"Wow, this feels so much better," he said.

"Okay, now try doing another pull-up."

Grant walked over to the same tree, grabbed the branch again, and pulled. This time he didn't hesitate, wince, or stop on the way up. His chin cleared the branch with ease, after which he lowered himself back down.

He looked stunned. "That felt fine," he said. "I can't believe it."

He wrote me later that week, letting me know he'd canceled his shoulder surgery.

The important lesson here is that his arms or shoulders were strong enough to complete a pull-up. Still, his tight fascia and other issues were making his arm and shoulder move unnaturally and painfully. Surgery wouldn't have fixed his shoulder. It *would* have left him mired unnecessarily in rehab with scar tissue that could have become its own problem over time.

Posture Is the North Star

My approach to how I treat individual patients is pretty simple. Posture is the foundation of everything for me—the North Star, as far as I'm concerned. Once that's squared away, I teach patients how to move more easily with their new and improved body alignment. Once posture and movement are both dialed in, the focus shifts to creating strong, resilient muscles. This methodology has allowed me to fix the most complex cases imaginable, even when a patient has already seen many other practitioners.

I break my approach down into what I call the three C's:

▶ Creation

▶ Control

▶ Capacity

Creation refers to methodically creating space or range of motion, ideally through manual therapy techniques and specific exercises.

Control refers to controlling this newly acquired range of motion.

Capacity refers to increasing speed, strength, power, agility, and endurance to enable better performance.

Traditional rehabilitation therapy tends to focus on one or maybe two of the three C's. Seldom does a practitioner look at all three components simultaneously while viewing posture as their North Star. For example, therapeutic massage, chiropractic work, and some physical therapy might focus only on increasing range of motion through soft tissue release and manipulations such as rubbing and cracking. Yet often, once the client returns to their regular activities, they have neither the control nor the capacity to prevent the injury from recurring.

Personal training usually focuses on strengthening, which is building capacity. But too often, this capacity is built on top of dysfunction. Creating a stronger muscle without the means to support it hardly seems like a recipe for success—more like a recipe for disaster. It's building capacity without the ability to control it. Imagine shooting a rocket launcher while standing on a raft in the water. Power is dangerous if you can't control it.

The goal of focusing on all three C's is to align a patient's body so that all of their movement primarily flows through their muscles. In this ideal scenario, the joints invisibly support movement. This flow-like state of movement can exist only when the joints are correctly aligned, a goal I'm always striving toward with my patients. I start with a strong foundation: a healthy and mobile system of tissues and joints, reinforcing correct postural alignment. Then I focus on building lasting control and strength, with a strong foundation underpinning them. I have no interest in building facades that hide run-down, broken structures.

Creating space by optimizing your body's posture, symmetry, and range of motion allows you to do any activity you want without fear of injury. Control and capacity will enable you to choose the level of intensity at which you perform your chosen activities. Think of the body's tissues (the fascia, muscles, bones, and nerves—all the elements we've talked about) as different instruments in an orchestra. Every movement is a different song. If each instrument can play only one note, there aren't many songs to choose from. Keeping each of these instruments healthy, with a wide array of notes to play, allows you to play as many songs as you wish.

Posture and movement are as personal as a fingerprint or signature. When I meet a patient, I begin by looking at their body's structure and how they stand and sit. This assessment lets me know how the person moves while highlighting areas of concern. Their movement patterns and posture tell a story, and the plot is how their past lifestyle choices and injuries led them to hold their body the way they presently do.

So many life experiences influence posture. Tall people, for example, often develop poor posture because the world wasn't made for people their size. Chairs, clothes, car and airplane seats, gym equipment—no one creates any of these things at scale for a target market of basketball players. So tall people wind up shoehorning their body into awkward positions, resulting in significant back and neck issues. Even something as simple as a conversation becomes tricky, with the tall person hunching forward and looking down at their counterpart to make eye contact.

Another group of people prone to posture issues is pregnant women. During the second trimester, as the fetus develops, the mother's natural alignment will change— the hips will go into anterior tilt and their center of mass will shift forward. The abdominal wall ends up being stretched as well and becomes less effective at helping you stay upright. Unfortunately, this position often leads to low back pain. To avoid this common pain in pregnancy, postural awareness is key.

I remember treating another guy, named Adam, who was self-conscious about his weight. He'd go around sucking in his stomach in hopes of hiding it. Over time his stomach flexing had caused back pain, hip pain, and other issues. I said, "I know sucking in your stomach makes you feel a little bit better about how you look, but it's terrible for your back, and it's not sustainable, you know?"

Only by understanding such patterns, formed over years if not decades, can I help someone. Treatment inevitably involves unraveling destructive patterns.

While I am carrying out these visual assessments, the relationships between various parts of the skeleton become clues in the mystery. How does the patient's rib cage relate to their pelvis? Is their pelvis tilted, and if so, forward, backward, or to the side? How does their head sit relative to their rib cage? What does their knee do when their foot hits the floor? Think of postural alignment and balance as dynamic, not static. We're not statues in the town square. Treating posture is treating movement, not correcting fixed positions.

I always try to instill awareness in a patient about what's happening and why. For example, when I say, "Have you noticed that you always lean to the right when you stand?" I'm pointing out things they might be doing, perhaps subconsciously, that are causing problems. I try to be their guide, helping them better understand their bodies so they can help themselves. It's the physical therapy version of that old saying "Give a man a fish, and you'll feed him for a day. Teach a man to fish, and you've fed him for a lifetime." The world will never have enough doctors and physical therapists to serve everyone individually. We need to help people live a better life by teaching them how to maintain their own bodies. I'm a firm believer that self-help can solve many current and future health issues related to posture.

Even minor changes can yield dramatic results. With their body's alignment "reset," patients can feel taller, breathe more deeply, and move more easily.

As I've already pointed out, most structural issues that prevent you from achieving a balanced alignment stem from things you've done to compensate for physical problems in your past, including injuries. Let's say someone badly sprained his right ankle when he was young. While healing, he started limping and bracing as protective strategies, even though his ankle swelled to twice its standard size. Simultaneously, his left leg naturally tried to do more of the legs' work, compensating for the right leg and ankle. It doesn't take long for this compensation to become an ingrained movement pattern. The human body develops more collagen to support whatever activity it performs, so in this case, the collagen thickens in the left leg, making it slightly stiffer. Once the ankle heals, this new movement pattern doesn't necessarily go away. Maybe the person starts running again. Only now he's running incorrectly because his body has retrained itself to compensate for the bum ankle, even though it no longer needs the protection. Once the right ankle is fully healed, he might have started having problems in his left leg, too.

That assumes his right ankle *did* heal, which is a big assumption. Often it won't. The person might find that long after the pain from the initial injury is gone, his right foot is stuck in pronation (i.e., flat feet), and his right knee tends to cave in at rest. In turn, this may have caused unevenness in his hips, which may have led to lower back pain. Of course, the person would have no clue his back pain started many years ago with a sprained ankle!

"I Sprained My Ankle Again, Vinh"

I witnessed an epidemic of this sort of thing during the pandemic, when our clinics were practically overrun with runners nursing sprained ankles. During the lockdown, everyone seemed to get into running. It made sense. You're stuck at home, sitting all day, and you want to exercise in a simple, cost-effective manner while getting fresh air and some sunshine and respecting the social distance required to defeat the virus. But one consequence of this increase in running was a lot of ankle rolls—when the planted foot twists outward or, more commonly, inward. And I swear, nine out of every ten people I saw who'd rolled their ankle had a previous history of rolling their ankle. So why did people keep spraining their ankles over and over again?

Unfortunately, nasty ankle injuries can change our gait due to the modified weight-bearing involved—the scenario described above. To correct the problem, a medical professional would aim to reestablish the full range of movement and to boost the ankle strength to its prior level. Easy, right?

In the end, a patient might say, "Well, I can walk pain-free; I think my ankle is fine now."

Maybe, but maybe not. Let me explain using a music analogy. (I love music, by the way, so much that at one point, I considered leaving the rehab industry to pursue a career in music.)

Let's take the piano. Its sound is about more than just pressing down in rhythmic ways on eighty-eight keys. The strength with which the piano keys are struck, the key in which the music is played—both factor into what a piece of music sounds like. And behind them lies the strength of the musician's knowledge: their ability to read musical notes, understand the influence of keys and scales, timing, and so on.

Our body is an instrument, too. But what influences its "sound"? A key modulator is the central nervous system. It allows us to create the space needed to move, to control that movement, and to define the capacity of our body to move.

If you don't play the piano for a while, you can't just pick up where you left off on a song you were practicing before you stopped playing three or six months ago. The tension of the strings will change, so you need to tune them, allowing the harmony of each string to flow together. Similarly, you need to "re-tune" your central nervous system after an ankle injury, not just heal the ankle. It's one thing to regain pain-free movement and restore ankle strength. It's another to train the ankle under all the circumstances that will challenge its capacity.

Proprioception refers to the body's ability to identify where it is in space. It is your sense of self-movement and awareness of your body's position. Close your eyes for a second. Touch your nose. You can do it because your body and brain have a sense of where your nose is in space. Our muscles, tendons, and joints contain the neurons (proprioceptors) responsible for proprioception, so you can imagine that an injury to these connective tissues might affect our body's awareness of itself in space.

It turns out that an injury can change proprioception. Remember the ankle rollers? They were almost all repeat customers. Sure, after the first injury, their swelling went down in due course, their range of motion came back, and their ankle felt strong. Walking became pain-free again. But why did their ankle roll again? Maybe it wasn't trained for running conditions. Perhaps using pain as the only recovery gauge wasn't enough. What was the capacity of the joint? Could it handle single-leg balance? Could it handle single-leg jumps forward, backward, and side to side? Could it do all that with the runner's eyes closed?

Well-trained rehabilitation specialists won't just declare an area of the body healed after the pain diminishes. They'll know that they must address proprioception in order to permit injured athletes to return to their functional goals. They'll know that the control and capacity of an injured area need to be challenged—the fine-tuning, as it were.

DO THIS NOW: Stand on one foot and try to do ten heel raises with your eyes open. Now do the same number using the other foot. Now repeat both sides, but this time with your eyes closed. No cheating!

Notice anything? Did you lose your balance before ten reps on either leg? Were you wobblier on one side than the other? Did it get more challenging with your eyes closed? If you answered yes to those questions, you might have poor proprioception, particularly regarding the leg that struggled more than the other. If that's the case, do these calf raises with your eyes closed.

If you feel wrong, you will likely move wrong. "Wrong" in the case of those ankle-rolling patients was *not* retraining their ankle's capacity to handle the demands of running, which ignited a cascade of complications that threatened to become neurological issues.

Good postural habits also benefit from proprioceptive training. Research has shown that proprioceptive input at the trunk and hips can influence how we sit, stand, and walk. Repetition of the exercises in chapter 6 will facilitate proprioceptive factors that provide constant neural input for solidifying good postural habits, help prevent injury in good postural positions, and challenge the body to maintain good posture in all settings.

My exercises will help you do three things with your movement and posture:

1. Create more space at various joints in your body. The ankle roller will have a full range of movement, and the person who sticks their head forward will get themselves back to an optimal curve at the neck, back, and hips.

2. Control this newly found space. The ankle roller can do single-leg calf raises, and the person that previously stuck their head too far forward now has the trunk strength to maintain this posture while working.

3. Challenge the capacity of this newly created space. The ankle roller can now control their ankle range and strength without looking and on different surfaces. The person with stronger, better alignment can apply this to driving, walking, and everything in between.

DO THIS NOW: Visit myodetox.com to start learning more about your body and futureproofing it. We have a blog with dozens of posts covering a range of physical therapy issues, rehabilitation, and futureproofing your body. I contribute some of the posts, but the majority are from other Myodetox therapists. You'll also find links to our social media channels, which are jam-packed with great information.

Seeing for Yourself

Unfortunately, I can't see each of you in person, so I'm going to point out ways that you can self-assess and determine what exactly you need to work on. The basic hygiene plan is suitable for everyone, but everyone is different, and some adjustments should be made based on certain conditions.

We constantly judge the bodies of others, but when was the last time you gave yourself the same level of scrutiny? Most people pay attention to their body only when it hurts or isn't working correctly. Otherwise, we tend to stand and sit on autopilot. I'm challenging you to pay closer attention to your body, to slow down and begin noticing not only the bad but also the good.

VIEWING YOUR BODY IN SPACE: A HANDY GUIDE

As you proceed through the book, you'll read a lot about how physical therapists like me view and talk about the human body. It's information you'll need to know to take full advantage of the advice I give you in subsequent chapters. Don't be intimidated by the terminology; it's not as complicated as it sounds. But it can help you futureproof your body.

Orientation Terms

ANTERIOR VIEW: the body as viewed from the front (Figure 5.1)

POSTERIOR VIEW: the body as viewed from the rear (Figure 5.2)

LATERAL VIEW: the body as viewed from the side (Figure 5.3)

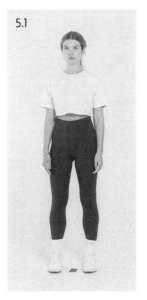

Anterior view

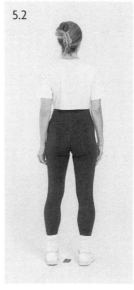

Posterior view

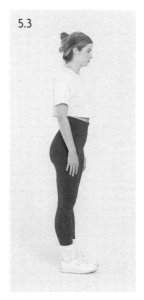

Lateral view

Planes of Movement

Movements of joints occur on different planes of the body:

SAGITTAL PLANE: cuts the body into left and right halves. Movement forward and backward occurs in this plane (Figure 5.4).

FRONTAL PLANE: cuts the body into front and back halves. Movement side to side occurs in this plane (Figure 5.5).

TRANSVERSE PLANE: cuts the body into top and bottom halves. Rotation and twisting movements occur in this plane (Figure 5.6).

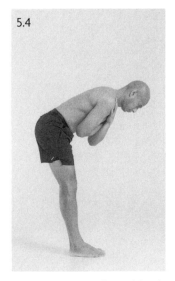
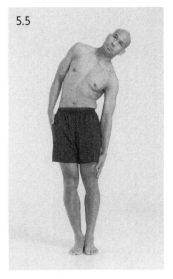
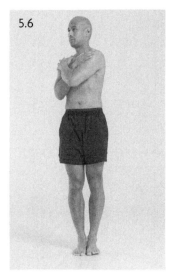

Sagittal plane—forward bend   *Frontal plane—side bend*   *Transverse plane— trunk twist*

To return to a better baseline, you may need to do corrective work based on a visual assessment, one you can easily do yourself. Selfies can also help identify less-than-ideal habits. Assessing your posture might seem intimidating at first. With a bit of guidance, though, you'll find it much simpler than you think. A mirror will suffice; better yet, have someone take three photos showing your body from the front, back, and sides. Wear as little as you're comfortable wearing and stay in the same spot with the same lighting for all three photos. The goal is to capture your body from head to toe.

HOW TO CAPTURE YOUR POSTURE WITH AN IPHONE

1. Put your phone on selfie mode.

2. Set up your phone at table height (Figure 5.7).

3. Take two steps away from the table. Put a piece of tape on the floor in between your feet. When you look back at the phone, your entire body, head to toe, should be in the frame of the photo (Figures 5.8, 5.9, 5.10).

4. Go back to your phone and set the timer to ten seconds (Figure 5.11).

5. Go back to the piece of tape and face the camera (Figure 5.12). Repeat and face away (Figure 5.13). Repeat and face to the left side (Figure 5.14). Repeat and look to the right side (Figure 5.15).

To draw a plumb line on your photo on iOS:

1. Open a photograph. Go to Edit.

2. Go to the top right corner to ". . ."

3. Choose Markup.

4. Choose the "Ruler" function on the bottom right.

5. Reposition the ruler to 90 degrees vertical (with two fingers).

6. Drag the ruler to (Figure 5.18):

- ► *Front view:* belly button

- ► *Side view:* greater trochanter

- ► *Rear view:* in between the PSIS (dimples)

7. Draw a line using the ruler.

We're not aiming for perfect symmetry here. No one on earth is perfectly symmetrical. When viewing yourself from the front, whether in the mirror or via a photo, the first thing to pay attention to is your body's left/right, upper/lower symmetry. For assessment purposes, visually split your body into halves, vertically and horizontally. When viewing yourself from the rear, photos will be more helpful than the mirror.

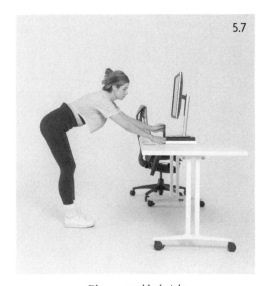

Phone at table height

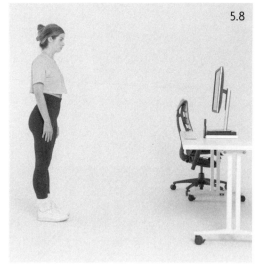

Two steps back, entire body visible

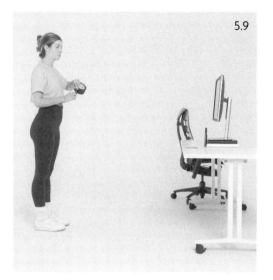

5.9

Tape setup

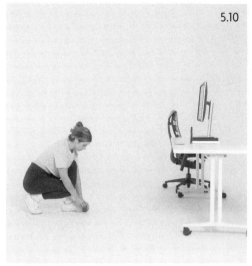

5.10

Tape placement for reference

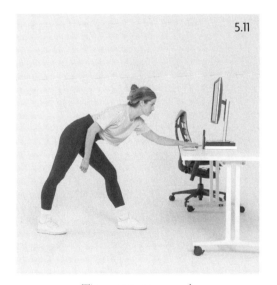

5.11

Timer set to ten seconds

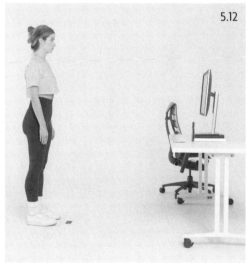

5.12

Facing the camera for front view

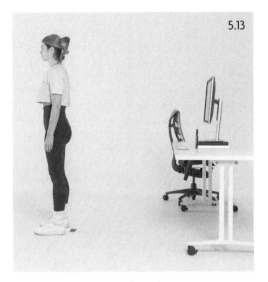

5.13

Facing away from the camera

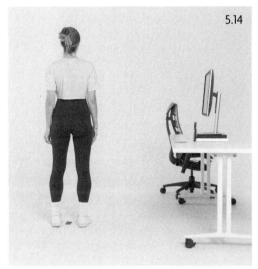

5.14

Facing to the left

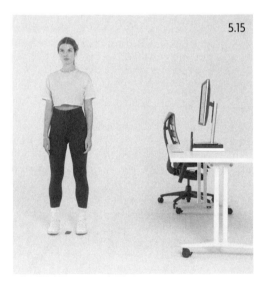

5.15

Facing to the right

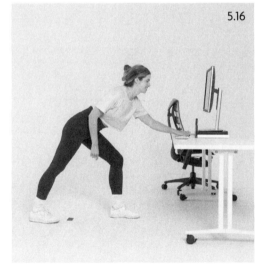

5.16

Check your selfies!

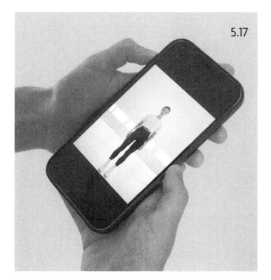

Checking the selfie

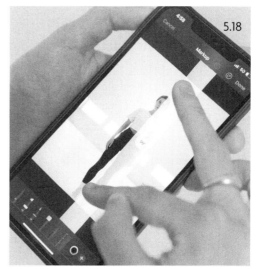

Plumb line placed on phone using "ruler"

When looking at yourself from the front or back, ask yourself these questions:

▶ Is my neck tilted or bent to one side?

▶ Am I rotated to one side?

▶ Is one of my shoulders elevated relative to the other? Is one more rounded than the other? Does one or both of my shoulder blades stick out from the back?

▶ Is my rib cage flaring out? Is it collapsed on one side?

▶ Does my upper body look like it belongs with my lower body? Do I notice a shift to one side versus the other?

▶ Is one hip higher than the other? Is it more rotated on one side?

▶ Do my knees touch together while I stand? Is one knee more collapsed than the other?

Next, turn your attention to the side view. This view should be compared to an imaginary line, called the plumb line, passing through the earlobe, the middle of the shoulder, the hip joint, the thighbone, slightly in front of the knee joint, and slightly in front of the lateral malleolus—that bony thing on the outside of your ankle. A posture that deviates away from the plumb line, along with asymmetries, may lead to muscular tension, pressure on the spine, decreased flexibility, joint problems, and impaired digestion and breathing.

So the plumb line should be your point of reference when asking yourself these questions:

- ▶ Is my head more forward than it should be?

- ▶ Are my shoulders more forward than they should be?

- ▶ Is my middle back (the thoracic spine) more rounded?

- ▶ Is my stomach sticking out from the plumb line?

- ▶ Is my pelvis rotated forward or backward? (This can be noted with your stomach very far forward, your buttock sticking too far back, or your tailbone feeling "tucked in.")

- ▶ Are my knees slightly bent?

- ▶ Are my feet flatter or higher on one side than the other?

To get a sense of where you may be experiencing restriction, here are a few tests you can do to assess your problem spots, from head to toe. You should use these as a before-and-after with the posture hygiene plan in chapter 6 and foam roll protocols in chapter 7.

NECK: Sitting or standing tall, bring your nose to the sky and then toward your chest (essentially looking up and then down). Reset, then turn your head to the right and to the left (as if you're checking something on your shoulder). Note which side you feel stiffness or pain while moving. For example, when turning your head to the left, you may feel tightness on the right side of your neck, or stiffness on the left side of your neck.

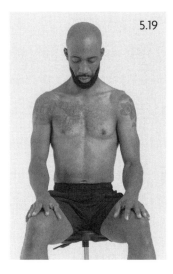
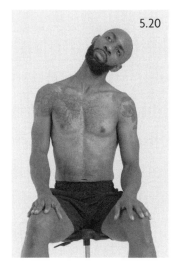
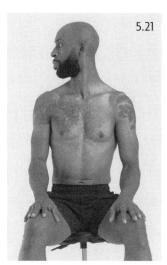

Neck movement

MID BACK: Sit down, with your hands crossed on your chest. Leading with your shoulders, turn to the right, with your head following in the same direction. Now turn to the left. Take note of any pain, discomfort, or stiffness felt with these movements.

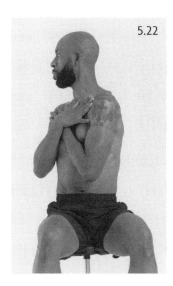
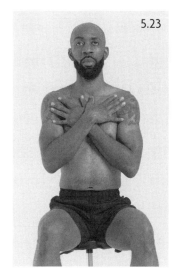
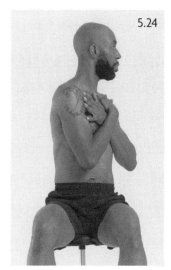

Trunk rotation

LOW BACK: Standing tall, with your feet together, make an attempt to reach for your toes. Take note of how far you can go before you feel stiffness or pain in your back or legs.

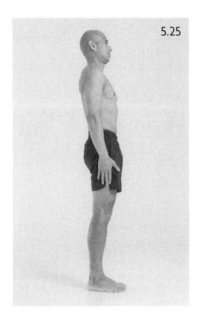 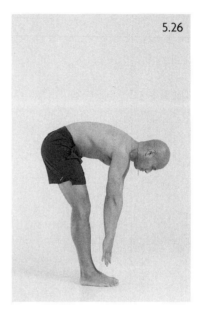

Toe touch

HIPS: Standing tall at first, with your feet shoulder-width apart, tuck your hips back in a squat, as though you are sitting in a chair. This means taking your hips from standing position and lowering them until you can't move any farther. The range of motion will vary widely from person to person and may reveal stiff and sore spots throughout the back, hips, thigh, knees, and ankle. Likely, this will be your most revealing test.

ANKLE: Standing six inches away from a wall, try to get one knee touching the wall without lifting your heel. Your hands and other leg can be used to support yourself. This is not a balance test. This is a test to get a sense of your ankle's available range of movement. Take note of stiffness or tightness you may experience in the front or back of the calf and shins. Make sure to perform for both your right and left foot.

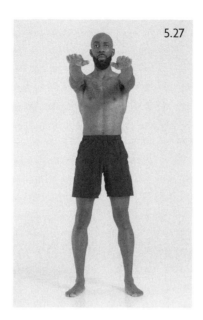

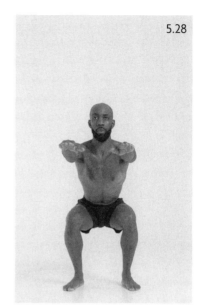

Squat

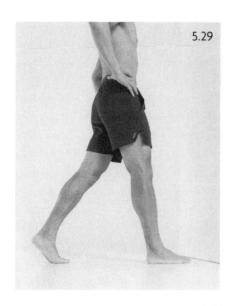

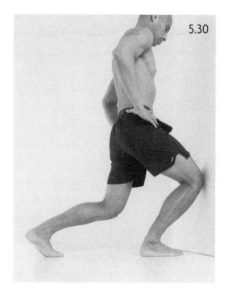

Ankle mobility

The Influence of the Pelvis

People whose pelvis tilts forward (anterior) tend to look like their butt is sticking out. The front of the hip rotates forward and down, forcing the back of the hips to rise. Using the plumb line, you can see how that anterior tilt increases lordosis (swayback) of the lumbar spine. When the lower back curves excessively, the stomach tends to protrude in response.

What happens to the *lower* body with anterior tilt? The hip flexors will pull the pelvis forward, leading to weakness in the abdominal muscles and glute muscles. Viewed from the front, anterior pelvic tilt typically causes the knees to cave in, placing more load on the inside of the foot, exaggerating a flat foot. The effects of the posterior pelvic tilt are the reverse of the anterior pelvic tilt. The point is to pay special attention to your pelvic alignment, as it can have an effect on your overall posture.

CONSEQUENCES OF ANTERIOR PELVIC TILT

If the pelvis is continually tilted anteriorly, the biomechanical result of this leads to the following:

1. Increased lordosis of the lumbar spine

2. Increased hip weakness and core weakness

3. Increased valgus at the knees (knees caving inward)

4. Increased pronation of the foot (foot becomes "flatter")

Usually, the anterior pelvic tilt will lead to an anterior shift of your center of mass—essentially, where your weight is placed with respect to your body. This configuration typically presents in an individual who is more mobile and has weak abdominals, increasing the risk of injury down the chain. To counteract this excessive mobility and core weakness, I usually recommend core work to help bring balance to the spine. An example of a great exercise would be a four-point plank.

CONSEQUENCES OF POSTERIOR PELVIC TILT

If your pelvis is continually tilted posteriorly, the biomechanical stress leads to the following:

1. Increased forward head posture

2. Increased thoracic kyphosis—that is to say, a more rounded back

3. Increased flexion at the lumbar spine

4. Increase in supination of the feet (arch of foot increases)

There tends to be increased tension at the glutes and hamstrings with posterior tilts, compressing the lumbar spine. This configuration is usually more stable, but this stability comes with a price: reduced mobility of the spine and feelings of overall stiffness in the back. To address posterior pelvic tilt, since it's more of a stiffness issue, a mobility regimen is usually what's needed. An example of this would be doing exercise 1 (gears).

6 THE POSTURE HYGIENE PLAN

LIFE MOVES FAST, and your body shouldn't slow you down. Just as you brush your teeth daily and maintain your car at regular intervals, your body must be maintained, or it will break down. The following daily regimen involves twelve exercises, many involving multiple muscle groups. This routine should provide nearly complete protection against posture-related ailments, just as daily brushing prevents dental decay and gum pain.

A NOTE ON CLOTHING: These moves are designed to improve your mobility and extend your ranges of motion, so wear something comfortable like shorts or sweats, which allow you to move freely.

A NOTE ON EQUIPMENT: None of the moves in the Big Twelve require any fitness equipment. A rolled-up towel helps for one variation of one exercise, but other than that, all you need is your own body and access to a wall and a table. Anyone on the planet can do this plan if they want to.

A NOTE ON WARMING UP: There's no need to warm up before you do this posture hygiene regimen; in fact it *is* the warm-up. While doing these movements you'll gradually increase blood flow throughout your body and promote natural lubrication around the joints, allowing your body to grow more elastic with each move.

A NOTE ON FREQUENCY: Perform this posture hygiene regimen at least once a day (although there's no reason you can't do it multiple times a day). By repeating these exercises, you're extending and maintaining ranges of motion, rewiring your nervous system, and changing your postural habits.

A NOTE ON PACE: You should aim for eight to twelve repetitions per exercise. Every repetition for each exercise should be held for one to two seconds (or one to two breaths). Your pace should be steady, deliberate, and fluid—neither too fast nor too slow. You don't want to be explosive in the same way you would be with CrossFit, sprinting, or plyometrics. Stay under control at all times.

A NOTE ON DURATION: Mobility training shouldn't take a ton of time, and my plan is no exception. The entire program that I've outlined here shouldn't take you more than fifteen minutes a day. As you get more familiar with the program, the program can be customized. You can start to focus only on the areas you feel you need to work on, essentially reducing your time spent to five to ten minutes.

A NOTE ON RAMPING UP: Trying to start this routine in its *entirety* is terrific but challenging. Many of you will find it difficult to learn one or two new exercises per session, so limit yourself to that. Start easy by doing only five minutes and committing to master the first two exercises. Then gradually add exercises as you get better. This will ensure that you don't bite off more than you can chew and that you can maintain a high standard of performance.

A NOTE ON MISSED WORKOUTS: If you skip this routine on a given day, it's okay. Expect some lapses here and there. Just don't give up. Eventually, you may have this routine so dialed in that you never miss a day. Be patient. Habits like this take time to develop, as we'll discuss later in chapter 11.

A NOTE ON SAFETY: To state the obvious, do not move into pain with any of these movements. You don't want to push your body past a point of mild tension or push through a range of motion that is not available. Lastly, keep your environment safe. If balance is an issue, have something nearby to grab onto or a chair behind you.

1. GEARS

(targeting the whole body—sixty seconds)

THE PROBLEM

Whenever I look at someone's posture, I focus on three areas first: the head, the rib cage, and the pelvis. This frame of thinking was inspired by the work of Gary Ward, a movement specialist whom I've looked up to and had the honor of training with. He taught me the importance of looking at the system as a whole, being aware of how major joints in the body can influence one another.

When you walk, your head and pelvis move together in the same direction, and your rib cage does the opposite. This dynamic helps drive you forward as you walk. These three structures are intimately connected. Unfortunately, if even one is out of whack, the other structures will struggle to deal with body alignment change. Like the gears in an engine that operate in pairs to transmit power to one another, the gears exercise operates to react and emphasize the relationship of the head influencing the rib cage, which influences the pelvis, and vice versa.

THE SOLUTION

The gears exercise involves the whole body. An excellent assessment tool, it's also a great exercise to help you achieve awareness and better ease of movement. As you repeatedly do this exercise, it will become smoother and smoother. When you are doing gears, the goal is to increase your body's ability to dissociate or separate. Hence the name gears—if you move one gear (the pelvis), the other gears (head and rib cage) must move, too.

The better you can do this, the more flexibility and muscular control you'll have. Everyday activities such as walking and running will become more efficient.

Lateral Plane (viewed from the side)

1. Stand straight with your arms hanging at your sides (Figure 6.1).

2. Begin by bringing your arms forward. Then, draw your pelvis back toward your spine, an action called posterior tilt. Your thoracic spine will flex or round, and your head will jut forward, the position many people end up in when they spend all day typing. You'll also notice that your feet supinate, and your knees flare slightly in this position (Figure 6.2).

3. Reverse this position by pushing your pelvis forward, an action called anterior tilt. Bring your arms back, palms up. You'll find that your thoracic spine will extend rather than flex, your chin will tuck, and your feet will pronate (Figure 6.3).

4. Move in and out of posterior and anterior tilt for a two-second count ("one-two").

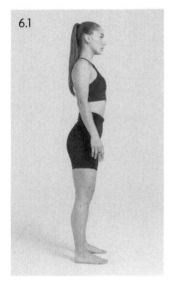

Start position

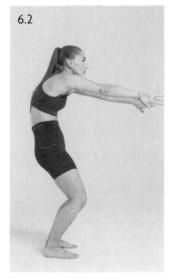

Posterior tilt of the pelvis.
Arms forward, thumbs down,
thoracic spine flexed.

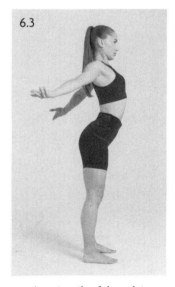

Anterior tilt of the pelvis.
Arms back, palms open,
thoracic spine extended.

Frontal Plane (viewed from the front)

1. Stand up straight, feet shoulder-width apart, arms hanging at your side, gaze fixed forward (Figure 6.4).

2. Lift (e.g., hike) your right hip. That's it. The only movement is lifting that right hip. As you lift, your trunk will sidebend right, and your head naturally will want to tilt to the left. Keep your head and neck relatively stationary, though, save for the slight movement induced by the hip raise. You don't want to be twisting or bending your neck independent of raising your hips (Figure 6.5).

3. Perform these in alternating fashion, one hip raise to the right, one to the left, and so on. Move in and out of each hike for a two-second count ("one-two") (Figure 6.6).

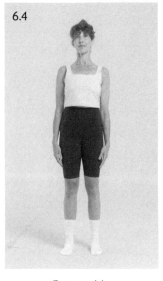

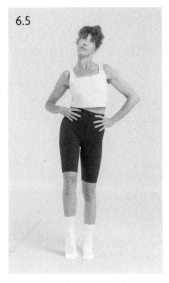

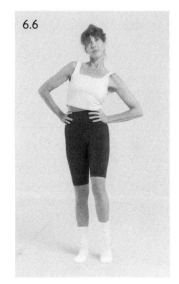

| *Start position* | *Right hip hiked* | *Reversed—left hip hiked* |

This move is also great for assessing which side of your hips is tighter than the other, as you alternate between the two sides. Follow my posture hygiene plan, and these sorts of imbalances gradually will even out. Don't worry if you lack perfect symmetry and perfection. I've been a physical therapist for fourteen years, and when I perform this exercise today, I still feel a slight difference on one side versus the other.

Transverse Plane

1. Stand up straight, feet shoulder-width apart. I like to keep my hands flat on my chest for this move (Figure 6.7).

2. Step forward with your left leg and simultaneously rotate your torso to the left (Figure 6.8). When you rotate, your head and torso go one way, and your pelvis will go in the opposite direction. That's what we mean by rotation. Make sure to align your head and torso. You don't want those going in separate directions.

3. After you've done one rep where your left leg comes forward and you rotate to the left, go back to the starting position and do the same movement; only this time, your right leg is leading the way by stepping forward (Figure 6.9), and you're rotating your torso to the right (Figure 6.10).

4. Continue alternating between legs. Move in and out of each rotation for a two–second count ("one–two").

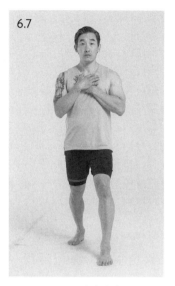

Start with left foot

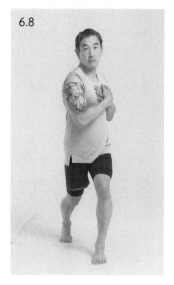

Left torso rotation

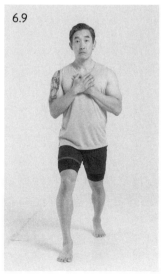

Start with right foot

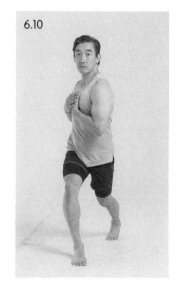

Right torso rotation

2. CERVICAL TUCK

(targeting the spine—thirty seconds)

THE PROBLEM

The neck is ground zero for posture issues. This intricate part of the human anatomy requires both stability and mobility. Achieving both capabilities requires the skull, seven vertebrae, and numerous muscles and joints within the neck to act in concert. Much of the movement begins at the base of the skull and the top two vertebrae, collectively referred to as the upper cervical spine. The two main joints that come into play are the atlanto-occipital joint (C0 to C1) and the atlantoaxial joint (C1 to C2) (Figure 6.11). Together, they account for flexion and extension of the head (e.g., nodding) and 50 percent of the neck's initial rotation. The remaining segments below account for the other 50 percent of rotation.

We've talked about tech neck, and this is where it happens. The more scientific description is too much extension of the upper cervical spine and flexion of the lower neck. This means that the skull base (C0) extends into the C1, which makes your chin poke out. (C1 to C2 doesn't extend because it is primarily concerned with rotation.) This position creates a lot of neck strain.

6.11

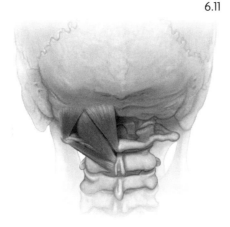

Muscles at base of skull

THE SOLUTION

The best way to fix tech neck is a simple chin tuck to strengthen and lengthen the muscles at the base of your skull and in the core of the neck. Version 1 is the simplest:

1. Sit in a chair with your back straight, knees bent 90 degrees, feet flat on the floor, gaze fixed forward (Figure 6.12).

2. Gently pull your chin back toward your cervical spine for two seconds (Figure 6.13).

3. Once you've come back as far as you can, slowly bend your neck to bring your head back, like you're watching a plane take off.

4. Focus on the movement happening in the cervical spine at the base of your neck.

5. Once your head is as far back as it can comfortably go, hold the position for three seconds (Figure 6.14).

6. Reverse the movement for two seconds to return to the starting position.

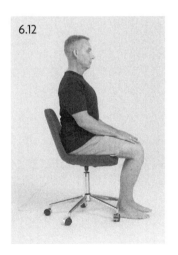
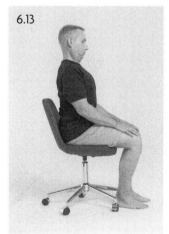
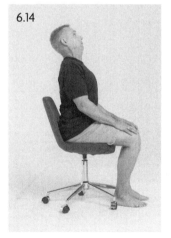

When this one gets too easy, try Version 2.

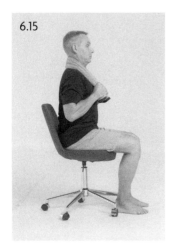
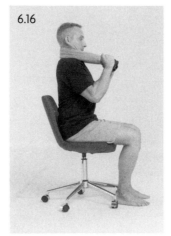
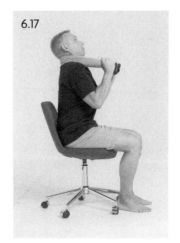

3. TYPE 1 AND 2 THORACIC ROTATION

(targeting the thoracic spine—sixty seconds)

THE PROBLEM

If you sit a lot for work or, like me, worked way too much on the couch at home during quarantine, your thoracic spine is likely stiff as a board. The thoracic spine consists of twelve vertebrae that lie between the cervical and lumbar regions. The middle thoracic spine stems from your neck's base down to the middle of your shoulder blades. It's a common source of pain and tightness for slouching desk jockeys.

The most common source of pain in this region stems from postural kyphosis, meaning the middle spine is overly curved and rounded. Kyphosis is a significant contributor to forward head posture and upper-crossed syndrome. "Upper" refers to the upper body, namely the neck, upper back, chest, and shoulders. "Crossed" refers to the X pattern of overused and underused muscles when viewing the body from the side. This pattern is caused by the posture I've discussed: rounded shoulders, head out in front of the torso, neck and upper back curved. Often the arms track forward a bit rather than hanging straight down. The net result is weak upper back muscles and tight neck and chest muscles.

The thoracic spine is already the least flexible area of the spine because it attaches to the ribs so, if you want to increase thoracic spine mobility and flexibility, pay equal attention to the rib cage.

A flatter thoracic spine (hypokyphosis) leads to excess pull of the neck extensor muscle group, resulting in overuse and possible spasms. The natural thoracic kyphosis of the back allows for efficient use of the thoracic erector muscles, providing a mechanical advantage to the curved spine. However, if this curve is absent (as seen in someone with hypokyphosis), this can stress the spine. But what if the curve at the thorax is too curved? This position is known as hyperkyphosis. In this position, your rib cage will collapse, causing your abdominal muscles to become shortened and tight. Consequently, your head will be pushed forward, leading to a hunchback-type look.

Thoracic spine dysfunction can contribute to:

▸ Neck pain

▸ Low back pain

▸ Poor shoulder mechanics and pain

▸ Thoracic outlet syndrome (pain, numbness, tingling, and weakness caused by compression between the upper chest and lower neck)

▸ Inefficient breathing

▸ A slouched appearance

Functionally, the thoracic spine allows for bending forward (flexion) and backward (extension) at the middle back. It's pivotal for moving your arms overhead, like going for a rebound on the basketball court and pulling the ball down to chest level. But if the thoracic spine isn't well maintained, issues can develop quickly.

The thoracic spine also allows for a certain amount of twisting to either side, called rotation. That's important because you can't maximize flexion simply by bending forward and backward. The thoracic spine needs to rotate a bit during flexion and extension, as well, to achieve its complete range of motion. It's a good thing, too, because that's how life happens: unpredictably along different planes and in different directions.

THE SOLUTION

Very few people work the thoracic spine through a full range of motion and through multiple planes. That's why I've chosen a movement exercise that will not only flex and extend your thoracic spine but also rotate it. Here's Version 1:

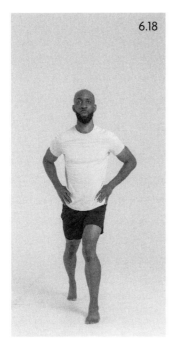
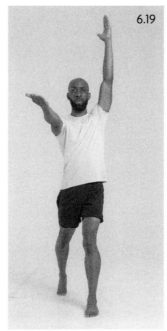
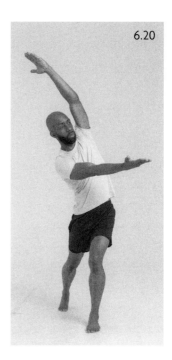

1. Start with left rotation. Assume a split stance, with your left leg in front of your torso and your right leg trailing (Figure 6.18).

2. Raise your left arm straight up toward the ceiling. Stick your right arm straight out in front of you, palm up (Figure 6.19).

3. Bend to the right, so your right arm begins moving across your body while remaining straight—this will lead to you rotating left. Don't bend that elbow. Lean into the movement with your hips. Move in and out of each rotation for a two-second count ("one-two") (Figure 6.20).

4. After performing ten reps, switch positions so that your right leg is forward and your left leg trails. Now your right arm should point straight up, and your left arm should extend straight in front of you.

5. Bend to the left, so your left arm begins moving across your body while remaining straight. Again, don't bend that elbow.

In Version 2, both arms move in the same direction:

1. Assume the split stance, your left leg forward, right leg trailing (Figure 6.21).

2. Keeping your arms straight, drop them down toward your right leg, then sweep them up and over your left shoulder, as if you were reaching down to grab something and then lifting it diagonally over your shoulder (Figure 6.22).

3. Complete ten reps, switch positions, and do the same number of reps.

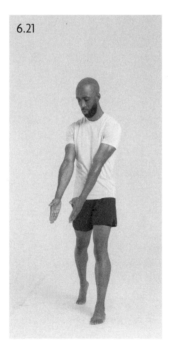
6.21

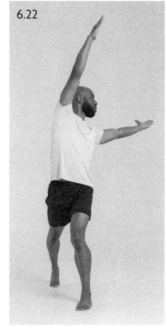
6.22

4. DYNAMIC LAT STRETCH

(targeting the lats—sixty seconds)

THE PROBLEM

Ever wonder why the back of Olympic swimming legend Michael Phelps had such a wicked V shape? You're looking at the epitome of well-developed latissimus dorsi muscle, aka the lats. This broad back muscle tends to be highly developed in swimmers, weightlifters, and climbers. The lats are responsible for pulling objects toward your body.

But did you know this muscle can affect your ability to lift your arm optimally? The length of the lats can significantly influence the extent to which your arm can elevate. Take swimmers, for instance: If their lats are tight, they won't be able to generate sufficient force for their shoulder. They could even develop a shoulder pathology. Add this to a slouched back, and you have compromised shoulder mechanics. Doing this dynamic exercise will help warm up and optimize your shoulder movements.

THE SOLUTION

This exercise is for the lats, but you should feel the stretch all the way from your hips to your shoulders when performed correctly:

1. Stand facing the edge of the chair or table in a crouched position, bent slightly at the knees and more prominently at the waist.

2. Reach across your body with both hands to grab the outer edge of a table or chair (Figure 6.23). Hinge at your hips by driving your buttocks back as you sink into the stretch.

3. To stretch the right lat, continue holding the table or chair with your right hand, and shift your weight to your right hip. As you perform this motion, your left leg naturally will straighten, while your right leg will bend even more as you sink into the right hip.

4. When you can't lean any farther to the right hip, take your left hand, and thread it through to the right (Figure 6.24). Your head will face toward your right. Hold for three seconds.

5. Return to the starting position and repeat. You should move in and out stretching the lats for three-second holds, ten repetitions, and three sets.

6. Switch sides, grabbing the other end of the chair or table with your left hand. Do the same number of sets and reps—three-second holds, ten repetitions, three sets.

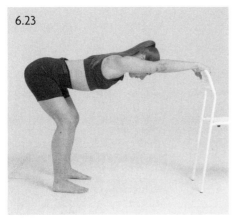
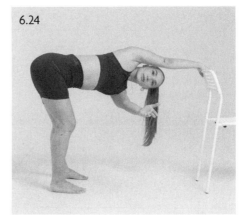

Both lats being stretched   *Focused on stretching the right lat*

The lats are a large muscle group, so you have two options regarding exercise tempo. One option is more sustained, where you do three to five reps of thirty-second holds per side. Another option is moving in and out of the motion in a controlled manner for ten reps, making this movement a little more dynamic.

By the way, these are awesome warm-ups for any pulling workout like rows and pull-ups.

Variation

To make the movement more difficult, while you're holding the chair or table with your right hand and sinking your hips to the right, bring your left arm under your torso in a scooping motion.

5. LATERAL BENDING

(targeting the lumbar spine—sixty seconds)

THE PROBLEM

I've already explained how the lumbar spine curves in the opposite direction of the thoracic spine above it. A common source of back pain and injury, the lumbar spine comprises five vertebrae working together to achieve flexion, extension, side flexion, and rotation. Several muscles attach to the lumbar spine, which can significantly affect the positioning of the pelvis, thoracic spine, rib cage, and legs.

You may wonder, "If there's an upper-crossed syndrome, wouldn't there be something similar lower down?" Enter the lower-crossed syndrome, which occurs when you have tight erector muscles in your lumbar spine, weak abdominal muscles, a weak gluteus maximus, and tight hip flexor muscles. These imbalances in muscle tension and strength can lead to poor posture and even asymmetry between the two sides of the body. For instance, it's possible to have one hip that hikes up higher than the other, which is sometimes misinterpreted as a "leg-length discrepancy." Or you may have glute tightness, where the buttocks region feels limited in movement, not to mention stiff and painful. These imbalances can significantly affect sitting and standing posture. Particularly if you're active, imbalances in strength and length can lead to tension, weakness, or even pain.

THE SOLUTION

If there's a possibility of one side of the back/hips being different from the other, then it makes sense that movements to address regions of tightness should be compared to the unaffected side.

Test

1. Fold your body forward, attempting a toe touch.

2. Take note of any tension or pain throughout the movement.

3. Side bend and slide your left hand down to the outside of your left knee.

4. Take note of any tension you feel during this movement.

5. Repeat on the right side.

Now that you've tested which area is sensitive, here's the exercise to help. I like doing exercises with a split stance, mainly because it mimics walking. This particular move opens up the hips and glutes:

1. Step forward with your left leg to assume a split stance (Figure 6.25).

2. Shift your weight forward as you push your hips out to the left until you feel a nice stretch in your hips and glutes (Figure 6.26).

3. Return to the starting position.

4. Do ten reps before switching positions so that your right leg is now forward in a split stance. Do the same number of reps you did on the other side.

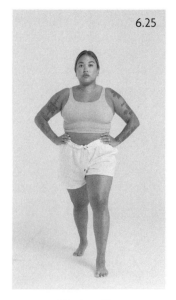
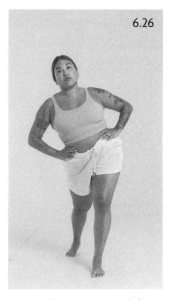
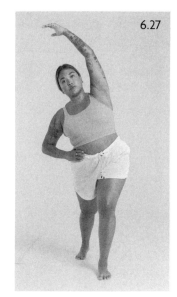

Start position

Pushing hips to the left

*Pushing hips to the left
with left arm elevated*

Variation

Using your left leg as the lead leg, place your right hand on your hip, raise your left arm, and arc it over your head as you shift your weight forward and push your hips out (Figure 6.27).

This will make the move a little more difficult. This stretch focuses on the hips, but you might feel it in your lat muscles or maybe the opposing adductor. Also, you'll probably notice that you feel this stretch more intensely on one side than the other. My hygiene plan should go a long way toward correcting that common imbalance.

6. McKENZIE EXTENSION

(targeting the lumbar spine and stomach fascia—thirty seconds)

The lower back is so important that it needs extra attention. Prolonged sitting leaves the spine flexed while shortening the abdominals and surrounding fascia. Even actions done with the best intentions can exacerbate this phenomenon. For example, the world went crazy when people erroneously thought they could get a six-pack with sit-ups. This oft-prescribed exercise had an unintended side effect: overly tight abdominals and fascia and a slouched torso, all risk factors for back pain. The most common position compromising the lumbar spine discs is flexion at the trunk and hips. Still think those sit-ups are good for you?

THE SOLUTION

I mentioned earlier that bending forward (flexion) is typically a stress position for spinal discs, particularly when they are unhealthy. It's only natural that exercises involving bending backward (extension) can help reduce pain while helping to reverse the disc bulge process.

Test

1. Keeping your feet together, your body upright, and your knees straight, place your hands along your lower back and bend backward.

2. If you experience back discomfort with this movement, note how soon you feel the pain.

3. After completing the exercise, retest your range of motion. You might be moving more with less pain!

This exercise is called the McKenzie extension, and it resembles the yoga pose upward-facing dog. It's meant to oppose the flexion stressors mentioned above and reduce or even reverse the bulge or herniation created from a disc exposed to excessive flexion.

1. Lie facedown with your hips hugging the floor and your forearms at your sides (Figure 6.28).

2. Gently push up with your arms while keeping your back muscles relaxed (Figure 6.29). Exhale as you rise. As you bend backward, your lower half should be relaxed.

3. Gently lower yourself back to the floor, with your arms doing most of the work.

4. With each rep, try to get higher without using your back muscles or hips.

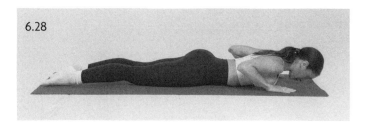

Start position

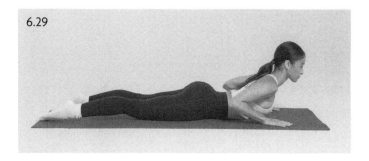

Pushing until restricted

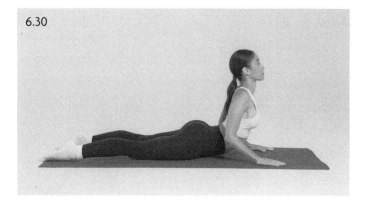

Variation for more range of motion

If you're stuck in an anterior pelvic tilt (i.e., your butt sticks up while you lie on your stomach), you're already in extension at the lumbar spine. It may help to place a pillow below your pelvis.

Variation

Not enough of a challenge? Fully straightening your arms with your palms down will lead to more extension and range of motion (6.30).

7. 3D PSOAS STRETCH

(targeting the hip flexors—sixty seconds)

THE PROBLEM

The hips are a critical area of the body yet are often overlooked, which is why I emphasize them so much. They lie squarely in the middle of the body and are essential for maintaining balance and stability. Pretty much anything you do in life requires healthy, functional hips. Tight and overused hips aren't just uncomfortable—they can lead to all sorts of other aches and pains, especially in the lower back. If they're not working correctly, you're going to see real declines in your performance and stability.

The psoas and iliacus, aka the hip flexors, are essential muscles affecting the lower back and pelvis. They attach to the front of the lumbar spine vertebrae and cross the pelvis to connect to the thighbone (femur). The hip flexors can become tight with prolonged sitting. And for those who have lost the connection with their core stabilizers, the hip flexors take on the role of "replacement core." Unfortunately, when these muscles stabilize the pelvis to excess, it pulls the lumbar spine and pelvis forward, resulting in an anterior tilt. That pinch in the front of your hips when sitting or squatting? The pain in your lower back when you're standing or reaching upward? It could all be coming from tight hip flexors.

THE SOLUTION

1. Assume a split stance, with your left leg in front of your torso and your right leg trailing behind. Focus on feeling a stretch in your right hip flexor muscles (Figure 6.31).

2. Raise your right arm straight up toward the ceiling (Figure 6.32).

3. Start shifting your body forward and allow your left knee to bend. Keeping your right knee straight (locked out), raise your right heel as you turn your body toward the left knee (Figure 6.33).

4. Reach for the ceiling with your right hand, feeling the stretch increasing in your right hip flexor.

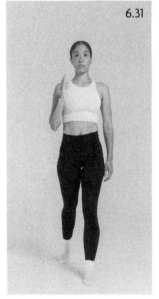 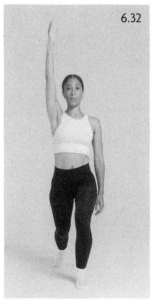 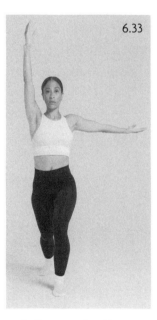 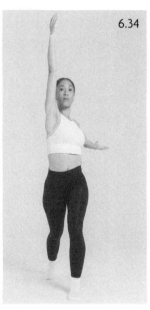

| *Start position* | *Right arm elevated* | *Left arm to the side* | *Variation—rotation added* |

Variation

Add a right hip drop and left torso rotation with your left arm outstretched to make it a full 3D stretch (Figure 6.34).

8. HIP STRETCH

(targeting the internal and external rotators of the hips—sixty seconds)

THE PROBLEM

Hip impingement often reveals itself in everyday activities like sitting and in athletic moves like squatting. The standard advice to combat this is to stretch the glutes. Unfortunately, many of these stretches don't address the real problem, which has to do with how the hips rotate.

It sounds complicated, but let me simplify it for you. When you stand and turn your feet toward the middle of your body (pigeon-toed), you rotate your hips internally. When you stand and turn your feet outward (duck-footed), you rotate your hips externally.

Hip impingement usually results from problems with internal rotation, and those glute stretches you've been doing don't really address that. In fact, medical professionals often use internal rotation to gauge possible trauma and damage to the hip joint.

THE SOLUTION

This hip stretch is meant to focus on improving your internal hip range of movement, minimizing hip pinching.

Test

1. Lying flat on your back, bring your left knee to your chest, aiming for your pecs.

2. Repeat with the right knee.

3. If you can move your knee close to the chest without lifting your back and feeling a pinch at the front of the hip, there's no impingement.

4. If there's some pinch, take note of the amount of range you have.

5. After doing this next exercise, retry the knee-to-chest test, seeing if the pinch is gone or if you can move your hip more without a pinch.

This exercise focuses on internal hip rotation:

1. Start by standing straight, feet shoulder-width apart (Figure 6.35).

2. Focusing on the right hip first, step forward with your left leg, turning your left foot inward so it lands at a 45-degree angle or thereabouts (Figure 6.36).

3. While your left foot moves forward and inward, rotate your torso 90 degrees to the right while bending your left knee and dipping your left shoulder while your right shoulder faces toward the ceiling (Figure 6.37).

4. Your right leg should stay straight. You should feel the stretch in the buttocks.

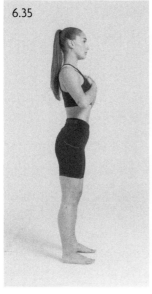
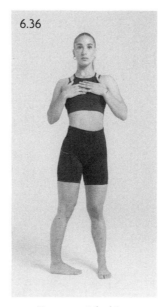
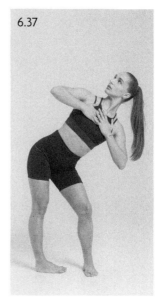

Start position   *Focus on right hip*   *Hips bent, torso rotated*

9. AROUND THE CLOCK

(targeting the lower legs—sixty seconds)

THE PROBLEM

Sitting in a slouched position places the pelvis in a posterior tilt. This may be influenced by overactive hamstrings, which may be linked to increased lower back pain. If you're a runner, you may be familiar with the importance of the gluteus medius (hip abductors) and knee pain. Still, runners can also experience increased activity in their adductors.

Let's take an even simpler example of how muscle imbalances can influence your daily life. Do you have a favorite leg to stand on? This seemingly innocent habit reflects an imbalance in the pelvis. It combines all the problems we've discussed above in one movement: leaning on one leg more than the other. In turn, the whole body compensates.

Test: Nothing fancy here. Walk around and get a feel of where you feel the tension in your legs. Maybe your quadriceps are tight, or one of your hamstrings is tighter than the other. I know I feel this after doing leg day! Retest yourself after this exercise by walking around again.

THE SOLUTION

Think of this exercise as using a clock:

1. Stand up straight with your arms shoulder-width apart (Figure 6.38).

2. Step back with your left leg to the six o'clock position and reach down to touch your right foot with both hands, keeping your right leg straight (Figure 6.39). Feel an intense stretch in your right hamstring? That means you're doing it right.

3. Return to the starting position.

4. Step back again with your left leg; only this time, it should land farther away from your body to the right, in the seven o'clock position (Figure 6.40). Reach down to touch your right foot with both hands. You should feel a stretch in the back and inner right leg.

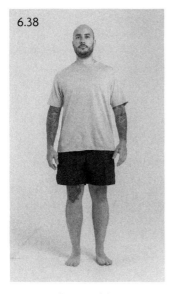

6.38

Start position

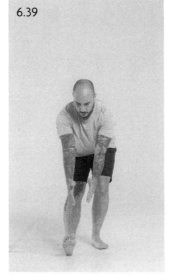

6.39

Six o'clock position

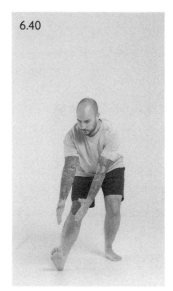

6.40

Seven o'clock position

5. Return to the starting position again.

6. Once your foot has come around to the nine o'clock position, lunge to the side (Figure 6.41). You should feel the stretch in your inner right leg.

7. Return to the starting position.

8. Move your right leg farther to the front.

9. The final position should lead to your right leg forward at twelve o'clock, with the stretch at the front of your left hip.

10. Switch positions and go through the same sequence, only this time with your left leg being the active leg.

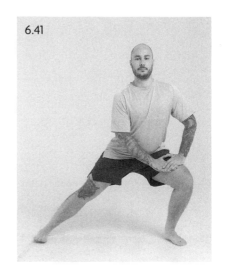

6.41

Nine o'clock position

10. SPLIT STANCE HINGE AND REACH

(targeting the posterior chain—sixty seconds)

THE PROBLEM

The posterior chain refers to the lats, glutes, hamstrings, and other muscles on the back side of the body. They work together to control hinging, pulling, and lifting motions. The posterior chain also plays a massive role in locomotion, providing the propulsive force during walking and running. Strength and mobility in this region also relate to the prevention of lower back pain. Because the posterior chain is such a pivotal system, any malfunction is problematic. In particular, poor mobility in this group of muscles increases stress on the low back, often the chain's weakest link.

A dysfunctional posterior chain often will aggravate the sciatic nerve. Different layers of fascia cover this nerve, which can get stuck in the posterior chain's tight muscles, such as the piriformis and hamstrings. If you've experienced shooting pain down the back of your leg or tingling in your feet, chances are the sciatic nerve was the culprit.

THE SOLUTION

Test

Keeping your feet together, bend forward and try touching your toes. That's it. Get a feel for where you may be tight, which may be different for everyone. You might feel the tension in your middle back, lower back, or behind your leg—the posterior chain connects to all these regions. Once you complete this exercise, retest your ability to touch your toes. You may find yourself moving with greater range, less tension, or both.

This stretch works your posterior chain:

1. Begin in a split stance with your right leg forward. Keep both knees as straight as possible (Figure 6.42).

2. Bend forward at the hips. Reach down with both hands, aiming to touch your right foot (Figure 6.43).

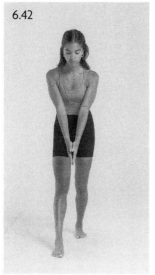
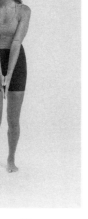
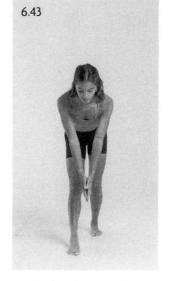
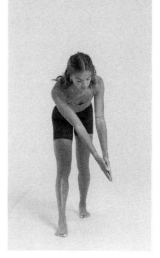

Start position   Twelve o'clock position   Eleven o'clock position

3. Do similar reach-downs fanning from the inside to the outside of your right foot. Use the clock analogy as a visual. Aim for the eleven o'clock (Figure 6.44), twelve o'clock (Figure 6.43), and one o'clock (Figure 6.45) positions of the front foot.

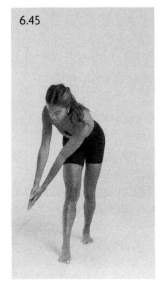

6.45

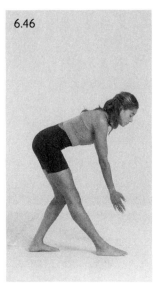

6.46

One o'clock position *Alternate angle twelve o'clock*

11. FOOT PRONATION AND SUPINATION

(targeting the feet—sixty seconds)

THE PROBLEM

Your feet are one of the keys to good posture, arguably the most overlooked factor. Each foot comprises twenty-six bones, thirty joints, and more than one hundred muscles, tendons, and ligaments, all working in a delicate dance to provide support, balance, and mobility. Paradoxically, the foot must be supple and mobile enough to absorb body weight (or multiples of it) thousands of times a day, yet firm and rigid enough to propel the body forward.

It may surprise you to learn that the foot contains more nerve endings per square centimeter than any other body part. The feet are sensory organs, feeding the body and brain with all sorts of important information and data.

The feet dictate how the body responds to the stresses of gravity from above and the ground below. The arches play a very important role in the structure of our feet and our responses to gravity and the ground. These arches are often described as being in supination (high arches) or pronation (flat arches). You don't want too much of one or the other.

Everyone can relate to how something as small as a pebble in your shoe can affect posture and gait. Even a grain of rice is enough to make someone limp. Now consider the thirty joints in our foot. If any are dysfunctional, even one joint can act like a pebble, influencing pronation and supination of the foot and affecting posture. Little wonder many people experience foot pain by the time they reach adulthood.

Part of the reason is that shoes worn in childhood force the feet into strange positions. From that point, footwear becomes less and less practical because of their ergonomic structure (take heels, for example). (I am a die-hard sneaker fan, so I find it painful even talking about heels.) Whether we have high or flat arches, we're often told to introduce something to our footwear that may alleviate dysfunction or pain (orthotics, anyone?).

THE SOLUTION

I can't tell you how many knee issues I've fixed in the past by prescribing foot exercises and by teaching people how to walk better. Teach your feet how to move well (pronate and supinate), and watch many issues, including pain, melt away!

Test: I just devoted a lot of words to the topic of feet, but the test for how your feet feel is simple. Walk around your home barefoot and get a sense of where you place pressure on your feet. Maybe you place way more weight on the heel of one foot versus the other. Maybe you walk on the outside of your left foot and the inside of your right. This walk is an excellent opportunity to get a feel for your feet. Once you've experimented a bit, retest your walk and see if you notice a difference.

Everyone needs to do the following exercise. It doesn't matter if you're high-arched or flat-footed. It doesn't matter if you love or hate cheese. (I hate cheese.) It doesn't matter if you like to put sauce on your food or keep it dry. (I hate too much sauce.) Exposing your foot to all ranges of movement is vital. Spend too much time in one region, and the opposite part becomes weak. Doesn't it make sense to expose yourself to your areas of weakness to improve your postural health?

Everyone's foot configuration is unique, so you'll feel tight in different areas. You also may notice that your left and right foot feel different when you do this exercise. That's okay. This exercise will help remedy any imbalance.

1. Stand up straight with your arms hanging at your sides.

2. Step forward with your left foot (Figure 6.47).

3. Bend your knee and drive it inward, which will flatten your foot. Your hips and torso should follow suit and rotate in the same direction as your bending knee (Figure 6.48).

4. On returning to the starting position, the opposite should occur: your knee, hips, and torso should rotate outward.

5. Throughout, you should feel a stretch in the bottom of your foot as you open up the plantar fascia.

6. Do five to ten reps per foot. Repeat twice. But consider doing this repetitively throughout your day, depending on your activity needs. Take your time and stretch out that tight feeling.

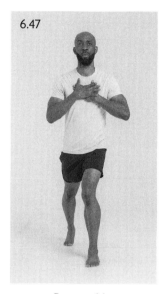 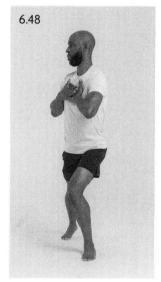

Start position   *End position*

12. BIG TOE EXTENSION + CALF STRETCH COMBO

(targeting arch of foot—sixty seconds)

THE PROBLEM

You've probably felt calf and foot pain after a long walk, a run (especially while exposing yourself to new surfaces and gradients), or jumping (anyone skip?). Sometimes this tension results from a condition called plantar fasciitis. The typical approach to treating this condition is specific stretches of the calf muscles. Though they may be involved with this tension, so is the big toe—the last joint affecting your ability to walk, let alone optimize your posture. But like I've said, the feet can heavily influence posture, and the big toe is no exception. If the big toe cannot extend sufficiently, this may lead to stiffness at the plantar fascia, and over time become plantar fasciitis. This could affect the foot, knee, hip, and more.

THE SOLUTION

Test: This one is simple. Standing straight, test one foot by trying to lift your big toe without moving anything else. Keep the balls of your feet on the floor. Some of you may notice your other toes move too, which is fine. Just keep the heel and balls of your feet on the floor. Once you do this exercise, retest your big toe movement:

1. Stand facing a wall and put the toes of your left foot up against it. The knee of your trailing right leg should be slightly bent (Figure 6.49).

2. Lean toward the wall with your left knee, which should produce a stretch in your toes (Figure 6.50).

3. Switch positions and repeat using your other foot.

4. You can shift and hit it from different angles, too.

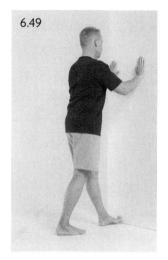

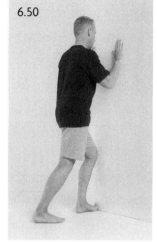

Start position　　　　　　*Knee to wall with toe*

Variation

Stand tall and lean your entire torso toward the wall. This action will stretch out your toes as well as your calf (Figure 6.51).

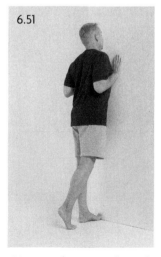

Variation for increased stretch

You might wonder if you should do these exact exercises indefinitely. Yes, you can. This isn't a bodybuilding plan, where the body will soon grow accustomed to the same movements and stop adapting as a result. These exercises will be effective as long as you do them. Now that I have said that, there's no reason for you not to add new moves to your arsenal periodically. I easily could give you ten different regimens to follow in sequence, but this book isn't an encyclopedia of mobility exercises and stretches. The moves I've chosen here are among my favorites, and time and time again have given the best and quickest results in my experience as a clinician.

If you follow me, Myodetox, or both on social media, then you know that we're always offering new exercises. Teaching has always been a favorite pursuit of mine. There's no greater joy than seeing the spark that goes off in someone's brain when they suddenly see the world differently.

The more you learn, the more you'll want to add variety, and you can do much of that on your own. Feel free to plug new moves into this routine or create entirely new routines. I encourage you to view this plan as a jumping-off point. Personally, I switch up my routine a lot. The more experienced you get, the more intuitive you can become with your exercise selection and programming. Along with working your body in new ways, switching it up now and then will help you keep your head in the game.

I hope that when you master this routine and the benefits materialize, you'll be inspired to share with others what you've learned. That's how movements begin. That's how influence spreads, and nothing would make me happier than to have readers like you become posture hygiene emissaries.

There's also a mental aspect to the routine I just offered. Practicing it gets you much more in tune with—and sensitive to—your own body. You're less likely to take it for granted. Even these relatively simple moves make you realize the extraordinary capacity your body has for movement. Some people go years without taking a set of joints and the surrounding muscle tissue through a full range of motion.

Because of that, they don't know what it feels like to move more effortlessly, more freely.

DO THIS NOW: Open your mind to the potential for self-transformation. When I was in college, I decided to be a singer, despite having no training whatsoever. I didn't even have any natural ability. Still, I went to a vocal coach on a dare from a friend and started learning. A year later, I was onstage singing and performing—if not brilliantly, then at least adequately. It might seem like that has nothing to do with developing great posture and warding off future health problems. But it does in the sense that it shows setting your mind to do something gets you most of the way there. Don't assume you can't just because you haven't.

And there's no excuse not to start now. You can spend a lot on your health and wellness, but you don't have to. It's more about prioritizing this regimen and finding time in your day—even if it's just fifteen minutes—to do it. Don't be afraid to practice what a sports psychologist friend of mine calls "appropriate selfishness," meaning sometimes you need to put yourself and your well-being first. If in ten years you're broken down or sick, you can't take care of your family anymore. So take the time to ensure that doesn't happen. Do the work necessary to feel better now and in the future.

7 FOAM ROLLING FOR NEXT-LEVEL MOBILITY

IF YOU'VE BEEN in a gym, a dance studio, or a yoga class, you've undoubtedly seen people working their muscles over these narrow cylinders. Since their introduction as a self-massage device in the 1980s, foam rollers have become a popular fitness and recovery tool.

You might wonder, *What does that cylinder do, anyway?* Foam rolling is a self-treatment tool that compresses tissues, mimicking certain benefits of a physical therapy session with someone like me. It employs a person's body weight to release painful knots in muscle tissue (aka trigger points), improve flexibility, extend ranges of motion, warm up muscles before a workout, and kick-start the recovery process after a workout ends. You don't need to be in pain to benefit from foam rolling, either. This is for futureproofing as much as it is for treatment.

I often find that people are good at foam rolling their lower body but have trouble finding effective ways to roll their upper body. But that doesn't have to be the case.

This section is an add-on to the Big Twelve if you want to achieve next-level mobility. When rolling an area, I recommend between thirty seconds and two minutes per roll. It often helps to do a second set as well.

How to Roll Your Calves

The calves run along the back side of the lower legs. To roll these muscles, your body should form the letter L when viewed from the side: torso upright (don't slouch) and supported by extended arms and palms on the floor, hands directly under your shoulders. Extend your legs in front of you, with one or both calves elevated and resting on the roller directly below your knees. Your toes should point up (Figure 7.1).

Begin rolling back and forth from the top of your calf to the midpoint (Figure 7.2). Your body will tell you when you hit a problem spot; when it does, sink into it and linger there until the pain or tightness dissipates a bit. Then keep rolling. Next, move the starting position to halfway up the calf, and begin rolling from there to the lowest part, near the ankle.

To change the emphasis slightly, point your toes inward or outward.

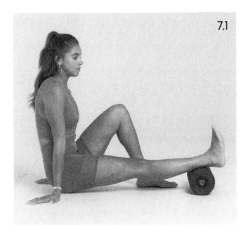
7.1

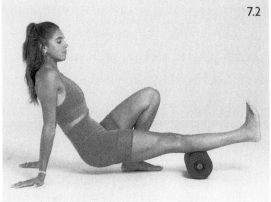
7.2

Variation

To make the sensation more intense, cross one ankle over the one on the roller. The added pressure allows you to dig deeper into the tissues.

How to Roll Your Shin Muscles

An essential muscle on the front side of the lower leg is the tibialis anterior, which runs along the shinbone. You may not have heard of this muscle, but you've probably heard of shin splints, a dull, nagging ache along the inner shin that tends to afflict runners. The tibialis anterior is the muscle that's hurting with shin splints. Although shin splints are seldom severe, they can lead to more serious conditions like stress fractures without proper treatment. It's your body's way of telling you you're doing too much, too soon.

The function of the tibialis anterior is dorsiflexion, the act of using your ankle to raise your foot toward your leg. To roll this muscle, assume the standard starting position of a push-up (Figure 7.3):

- ▶ Hands directly below your shoulders

- ▶ Palms on the floor for support

- ▶ Legs trailing behind you

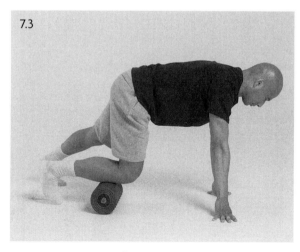

Start position

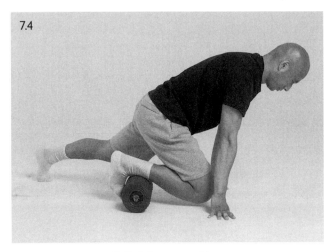

Rolled down to ankle

The toes of one foot should be touching the floor for stability, but the opposite leg should be elevated on a roller, with the point of contact being the top of the shin. Begin rolling back and forth at a measured pace, looking for tight spots and trigger points you can sink into and release (Figure 7.4). Turning your foot in either direction changes the emphasis and will bring more muscle and less shin bone into contact with the surface of the roller. You can probably roll the entire anterior tibialis without resetting your position, although if you can't cover the whole muscle, hit the upper half first, followed by the lower half.

How to Roll Your Adductors

The adductors are the five small muscles that combine to form the inner thigh musculature. Their primary function is bringing the thighs together. (Another set of small muscles, the abductors, move the thighs apart.) The adductors originate at the pelvic bone and connect to the thighbone, slightly above the knee.

Sit too much, and these muscles inevitably will tighten, risking groin pain and a reduction in mobility. Rolling can help remedy these adverse outcomes.

Adductors can be a little tricky to access because of their awkward location. In my experience, adductors might be the single most difficult muscles to roll. But if you position your body correctly, you can roll these tricky muscles.

To perform the move, position the roller perpendicular to your body, and then move toward one end of the roller so that one inner thigh is touching it and the other leg lies beyond it (Figure 7.5). Your elbows and forearms should be flat on the ground; the knee of the leg on the roller should be slightly bent, while the free leg should be pretty straight (Figure 7.6).

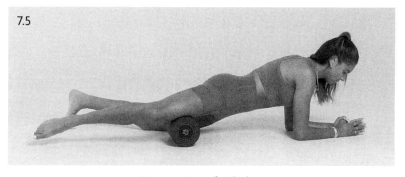

Start position of right knee

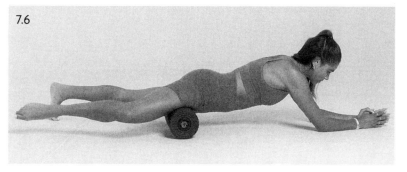

Foam roller near hip

Starting with the roller positioned directly above your knee, gently rock back and forth in the direction of your pubic bone. The roller should travel only six to eight inches. Next, position it above the uppermost point of the previous roll, and rock back and forth from there. It may take a third repositioning to reach to where the adductor meets the pubic bone. From there, gently rock back and forth over the upper inner thigh, up to where it meets the groin.

When you feel a pressure point or any sort of pain throughout the stretch, hold that position until the tension releases, even if it feels uncomfortable. However, stop if you feel numbness or tingling.

Whatever you do to the adductors on one side of the leg, perform the same action to the other side as well for the sake of balance.

Variation

To increase the bite on the adductor, use a higher-density roller, one with less give. To make it even more challenging, roll your adductors over a lacrosse ball or softball.

How to Roll Your Quadriceps

Next, I want you to roll your quadriceps, the large muscles covering the front of your thighs. Begin in a plank position, with your elbows and forearms on the mat or floor. Your legs should extend behind you, one or both of them elevated on the roller, with the point of contact directly above the knee (Figure 7.7). (You can roll both legs at once or do them individually; it's up to you. One leg at a time allows for more focus on any trigger points that might reveal themselves.)

Begin rolling your thigh back and forth at a measured pace (Figure 7.8). It doesn't have to be straight back and forth, either. Tilting your torso to one side or the other changes the emphasis, as does pointing your toes in either direction. Feel for tender spots and areas of tension; once you find them, spend extra time working on those areas. Sometimes I'll hold my position on a trigger point for thirty to sixty seconds. Get to the top of the quadriceps, too, and then back down to right above the knee.

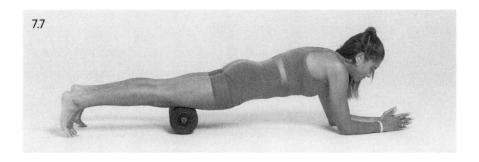

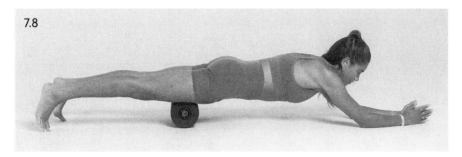

How to Roll Your Hamstrings

Do you constantly feel like you have tight hamstrings, and no matter how much you stretch, it never feels quite right? Foam rolling might help.

The most common knee injury strikes the ACL. If you want to protect your knees from this devastating injury, focus a lot of attention on your hamstrings, the large muscles on the back of the upper legs. There are three major players in what we call the hamstrings:

- ► Semitendinosus (medial)

- ► Semimembranosus (medial)

- ► Biceps femoris (lateral)

Having strong hamstrings improves your knee stability, protecting against excessive shearing and twisting. Unfortunately, the hamstrings are highly prone to tightening up, especially after long stretches spent sitting. Hamstring tightness limits the muscle activation.

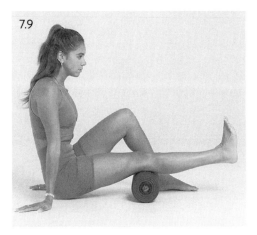

Start position

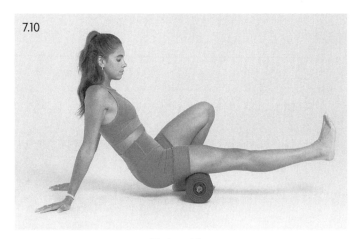

End position

To roll your hamstrings, sit on the floor or a mat with your arms straight, and palms on the floor supporting you. The roller should be under your legs, right above the knee (Figure 7.9). Your legs should extend straight in front of you. Roll halfway up the hamstrings and then back down to the starting position (Figure 7.10). As with the quadriceps roll, turning your toes inward or outward will shift the emphasis a bit, which I recommend doing. Again, you're hunting for trigger points. When you find them, focus on that area until any pain or tightness dissipates.

Once you're done rolling the bottom half of the hamstrings, reset your position so that the starting point is the endpoint from last time, halfway up the back of the upper leg. From there, roll up to the bottom of the glutes and then back down to the midpoint, continuing this back-and-forth motion.

How to Roll Your Glute Muscles

The gluteus medius lies in the outer buttocks region and plays a crucial role in pelvic stability and functional movement, particularly when standing on one leg. When the gluteus medius is too tight or weak, it can cause problems throughout the body, including knee pain. Foam rolling this muscle can release trigger points, allowing for more hip flexibility and mobility and a greater range of motion.

Roll these muscles one side at a time. You want to angle your body to let the roller dig deep into the gluteal muscles, and you won't be able to do that if the glutes on both sides are resting on the roller simultaneously. For the sake of this description, let's hit the gluteus maximus (largest glute muscle) on the right side first. Sit on the roller, supporting yourself with your arms extended behind you and your palms flat on the floor. The point of contact for the roller should be your right glute. Now cross your right leg over your left knee (Figure 7.11). Using your arms, you want to slightly push yourself forward, specifically rolling over your glute (Figure 7.12). You should note that the movement is quite small. If you need to maintain your balance, make sure to use your left foot for support.

As you roll, listen to your body; if you feel tightness or pain, linger on the spot for a while, holding it, gently rocking back and forth.

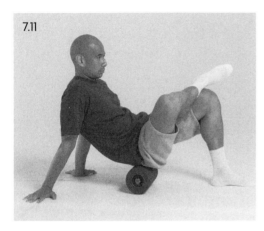

Start position

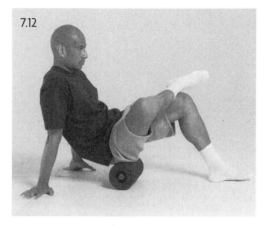

End position

Variation

To make this technique even more intense, use a lacrosse ball instead of a roller. The ball is harder and can dig deep into a given spot.

How to Roll Your Stomach

Everyone understands that they need to stretch their back, but rarely do people stretch their stomach area. That's an oversight. Your stomach tissue often gets tight and compressed over time due to long periods of sitting or endless sets of crunches. The foam-rolling goal is to open up the region, mobilize the spine, and release any trigger points or other tension. Not only will opening up your stomach tissue help you feel more relaxed overall, but it also might relieve some of your chronic neck and shoulder stiffness that you feel from working at the office all day.

Begin in a plank position with your elbows and knees supporting your body, and the roller positioned under your stomach as the point of contact (Figure 7.13). Slowly begin rolling up and down your stomach, directly below your rib cage to directly above your belt line (Figure 7.14). Go easy at first, especially if you've never rolled your stomach before. It's a sensitive area. If you find a tender spot, gently sink into it until the pain and tightness ease.

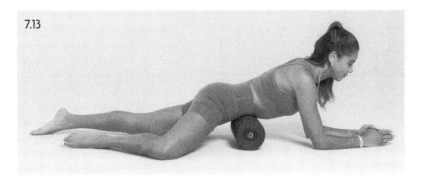

Above the belt line

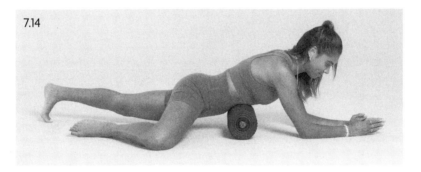

Just below the ribs

After finishing, stand up straight and take several deep breaths. You may find your breathing to be less restricted.

How to Roll Your Thoracic Spine

Sit on the floor or a mat with a roller behind you and your knees bent. Lean back until your back touches the roller; the point of contact should be just below your shoulder blades (Figure 7.15). Place your hands behind your head for support. Raise your hips off the floor or mat and gently roll up toward the top of your shoulder blades (Figure 7.16). Don't pull through your hands or move through your neck; your hands are there only for support. As you roll, feel for any tightness or pain in the region. If you find any trouble spots, stop for a moment and let your body weight and the roller sink into them. Sometimes this is all it takes to release pain points. Once you reach the top of the shoulder blades, reverse the motion and return to the starting point.

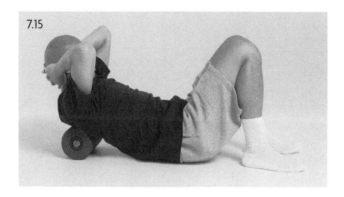

7.15

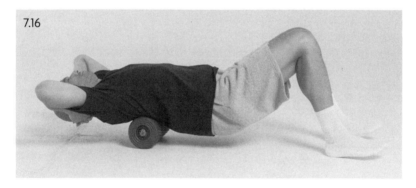

7.16

Variation

Bringing your elbows together will protract the shoulder blades and hit the thoracic spine slightly differently from the standard position described above.

Going from Single Moves to Combos

Now that you know how to foam roll, I'm going to show you how to maximize the use of the roller. To use a boxing analogy, I've shown you punching techniques; now I want you to learn the combos for a knockout.

We tend to think of our muscles acting in isolation. The biceps bend the arm, the quadriceps straighten the knee, and so on. But more complex movements require muscles to work together like an orchestra. For example, when you lift something heavy off the floor, you should use both legs to bend and both arms to pull. Try lifting something off the floor while balancing on only your left leg while using your left arm to pull the object. It's not easy. Now balance on your left leg and pull with your right arm. Much easier. This is an example of your myofascial sling at work. These slings comprise muscle, fascia, and ligaments working as one to create efficient mobility and stability.

Such slings are associated with large, dynamic movements. They work like an X: if the left side is working, the right side of the associated sling will work in sync. Therefore, when one muscle in the sling system contracts, the distribution of that force can be seen in another muscle. When tightness is found in one part of the body, there's likely tightness in another region.

I'm going to share several key foam-rolling combos that reflect the relationships created by these myofascial slings:

1. Calves: If either calf muscle is sore, roll both calves, both hamstrings, and the middle back.

2. Hamstrings: If either hamstring is sore, roll both calves, both hamstrings, and the middle back.

3. Shins: If either shin muscle is sore, roll the same-side shin, calf, quad, and hamstring.

4. Glutes: If either glute is sore, roll that glute and the same-side quad, as well as the middle back.

5. Middle back: If your middle back is sore, roll both quads, both hamstrings, both sides of the stomach, and, finally, the middle back.

6. Groin: If your adductor (groin) muscles are sore, roll both sides of the stomach and the same-side glute. For example, right groin muscle tightness requires rolling the entire stomach and the right glute.

7. Quads: If your quads are sore, roll the same-side shins, calves, and glutes. For example, right quad tension requires rolling the right calf, right shin, and right glute.

Foam rolling can be very effective in short-term pain management and freeing your movement. But its full potential can be realized by addressing other areas that contribute to the tension spot. Using this protocol, you can self-manage your pain spots by addressing other regions that you may not have realized contribute to your discomfort. You're not just learning to punch. You're learning the combinations for a knockout.

Choosing the Foam Roller That's Right for You

For such simple, lightweight, portable therapeutic devices, foam rollers come in a vast array of colors, shapes, surface textures, and sizes. Some models even vibrate.

You could try out dozens of rollers to find the one that works best for you, but I want to save you time and money. This quick guide discusses the different attributes of foam rollers and how they might factor into your purchase decision.

Density

Foam-roller densities range from rock-hard to squishy. As a rule, start with a softer roller and graduate to harder, denser models. Especially for newbies, the hard ones can be pretty painful at first. But as you grow more used to the sensation of the roller hitting a trigger point and other areas of myofascial congestion, you'll appreciate the effectiveness of the more rigid roller while experiencing less pain. The harder rollers tend to be more durable, whereas the squishier ones gradually lose their shape.

Length

Foam rollers can measure less than a foot to upwards of three feet. The lengthier models are great for rolling larger areas, such as the back, while the shorter ones work well for small, hard-to-reach nooks and crannies, such as the inner thighs. I recommend that a beginner who is buying a first roller choose a longer version.

Surface Textures

The surfaces of foam rollers also vary. Most rollers have a smooth surface, but some have a grid-type surface resembling tire tread. The smooth ones tend to be better for newbies because they are gentler and less expensive. The ones with more complex surface topography allow you to dig deeper into problem areas, but they can be more expensive.

Price

A foam roller needn't be a significant investment. Standard rollers run about $20, while models with fancy tread and vibrational capabilities can run $50 or more. You might start with a relatively inexpensive model; if you find it worthwhile, graduate to a more elaborate and expensive model later. Either way, foam rollers are an excellent investment in futureproofing your body.

8 TEN COMMON HEALTH AILMENTS SOLVED

I REMEMBER TREATING a female patient of mine, Sarah, in Toronto. She had been diagnosed with hip arthritis at sixty-six. She told me that her pain had developed over the year since she retired, and that this was now affecting her quality of life in retirement. So I asked her "What changed in the past year?" Because she was sixty-six, it made sense that her answer was: "I retired from working as a postal worker." So I followed up with "What have you been up to since then?" Naturally, she told me that she had been spending time with her grandchildren and trying to walk daily. I noticed that she had a smart watch—one that could count steps. So I asked her, "How many steps are you averaging?" She told me something that gave me a hint of her life since retiring: "Not nearly as much as I did working as a mail carrier. And now my doctor said my X-rays look like I need a hip replacement!" She exhibited pain at her outer hip and some joint capsule restriction consistent with hip arthritis, but no groin or middle thigh pain. Now, you as the reader should know that groin and middle thigh pain is a hallmark region of pain for hip arthritis, and this is typically felt in the morning and aggravated with activity. Interestingly, Sarah showed none of this. In fact, she felt better with activity. I told her something really simple: "Sarah, you gotta move. Your pain seems to have gotten worse with your not moving. Your signs and symptoms are consistent with immobility. You've had pain for only a year, but arthritis takes years! I don't think your arthritis is related to your pain." We worked on traditional strengthening together typically seen in outpatient rehabilitation: squats, lateral hip strengthening, etc. But I decided to challenge her mobility with the same exercises that are in this book: lateral bending (exercise 5), 3D psoas stretch (exercise 7), the hip stretch (exercise 8), and around the clock (exercise 9), to name a few. Of course we did these as safely as possible. Additionally, I asked her to increase her walking as much as she could. I'm happy to say that Sarah never had that hip replacement, and last I heard, she was still doing her mobility exercises.

With this plan I don't want to leave anyone behind, regardless of their starting point. I think my strong feelings about that have a lot to do with my Vietnamese heritage. We were raised to take care of others, especially the extended family. These days I take that impulse and broaden it to include caring for everyone on the planet, the family of humankind. Bruce Lee said it perfectly: "Under the sky, under the heavens, there is but one family." That may sound naively positive, but I firmly believe it. Certainly, Myodetox is a large and growing tribe of like-minded individuals. A family. A tribe. The MyoTribe.

So with respect to inclusivity, I wanted to make sure I touch upon common ailments seen in my practice, as well as how my postural mobility exercises can address them. They won't be cure-alls, but it's meant to give you a head start.

Some of you will come to this book plagued by an issue such as tendinitis in your knee or neck pain. I want to give you a way to deal with it quickly and effectively, so nothing stops you from following this overall posture hygiene plan. Of course, most—or perhaps all—of the conditions I'm about to match exercises to won't apply to you; keep going if they don't. But many of you *will* see certain conditions listed and think, *Aha, that describes me to a tee!* If so, slow down and listen up. Like my client, Sarah, you'll find that sometimes the best fix is movement itself. With the ailments listed below, my exercise plan will give you a head start and make sure these never become an issue for you.

As you go through the list, you'll see exercise numbers corresponding with each condition. These numbers refer back to the moves in the Big Twelve. If you have any of the conditions cited, find the associated numbers and do more of those movements to help address your situation or condition.

Ailment No. 1: Headaches

THE PROBLEM

We sit in the car, sit at our desks, sit to eat, and sometimes even sit to exercise. And when we're sitting, we're usually focusing our gaze on a screen. One consequence of this posture is a lot of people suffering from headaches.

Headaches come in several types, but two in particular are influenced by neck positions: tension and cervicogenic. Tension headaches are the most common stress-related headaches, and they involve the muscles attached to the neck and head (Figure 8.1). These headaches can be triggered by stress. They usually don't make you nauseous, but you might find it difficult to concentrate on a task when a tension headache is raging. Symptoms tend to reverberate on both sides of the head or neck and last from a few hours to several days.

Cervicogenic headaches are less common than tension headaches and tend to strike people aged thirty to forty-five years old. These typically involve the upper neck (the cervical spine) and the base of the skull. Importantly, cervicogenic headaches are aggravated by neck movement. Unlike tension headaches, cervicogenic headaches are often limited to one side or the other. In our

8.1

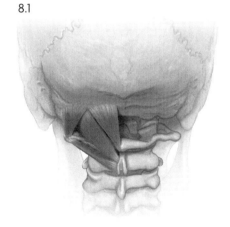

Muscles at base of skull

Myodetox clinics, we see a lot of these headaches ranging from younger patients who sit throughout the day (e.g., students and desk workers) to elderly patients who've sustained significant wear and tear where the neck meets the skull.

THE SOLUTION

Tension and cervicogenic headaches can be influenced by the neck, whose muscles and nerves are affected by posture. Specifically, increased time spent with a rounded mid back and chin-poked head can lead to tension at the base of the skull, leading to headaches. So to minimize the risk of tension and cervicogenic headaches, you want to understand two principles:

▶ Mobility at the neck and mid back can reduce headache risk.

▶ The positions you stay in (e.g., standing or sitting) can influence your headaches.

To address the neck and mid back, focus on exercise 2 (cervical tuck) for the neck and exercise 3 (type 1 and 2 rotation) for the mid back. Most important, spending time away from this posture is very important. Make sure you're attempting to stand after thirty minutes of sitting to reduce the risk of these headaches, and spend time doing my neck and mid back exercises. Additionally, you can foam roll your mid back for two to three minutes.

Ailment No. 2: Numbness and Tingling Down the Arms and Hands

THE PROBLEM

If you experience significant numbness in your arms and hands, along with chest pain and significant shortness of breath, head to the ER as fast as possible! It's imperative to rule out something catastrophic involving the heart. However, if you're feeling only a bit of numbness and tingling, immediately schedule a visit with a health-care professional to figure out what's happening. (If you want the best, visit one of my Myodetox clinics.) Whatever you do, please don't ignore it! Numbness and tingling seldom go away on their own, and they usually get worse.

8.2

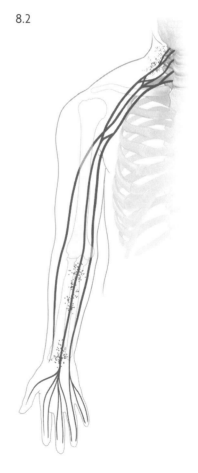

Earlier, I explained the relationship between headaches and neck muscles and how the latter are at the mercy of posture. Likewise, numbness and tingling can be influenced by neck position. We've talked about forward head posture, which typically leads to excessive flexion of the middle to lower neck. This may impinge on the nerves that emerge from the spinal cord to innervate the skin and muscles of the arms, forearms, and hands. This is why conditions like carpal tunnel syndrome and thoracic outlet syndrome can manifest from the neck. That's how neck posture can cause numbness and tingling.

THE SOLUTION

Numbness and tingling down the arm will often manifest due to compression in some region along its pathway. Regardless, focusing on the mobility of your nerves is key. Neurodynamics refers to the relationship between the mobility of our nerves and musculoskeletal system. A healthcare professional (e.g., physical therapist, chiropractor, or physician) can help you determine which specific nerve is involved with your pain and tingling, but particular exercises in my book can also help—both to address these nerve problems and ensure they never come back.

Additionally, you'll want to focus on your posture, which is the basis of the exercises I've provided. If you're rounded at your mid back, with your head too far forward, you're more susceptible to numbness and tingling. Steer clear of things that tend to crank your neck forward such as sleeping with too many pillows, jutting your neck forward when you're lifting weights, and looking down at your phone constantly.

Here are a few things you need to consider if you're experiencing numbness and tingling:

- ▶ If you're noticing that a particular position aggravates your numbness and tingling, you need to immediately identify this position and avoid it as much as possible.

- ▶ Understand that to improve your neurodynamics, you'll need to maximize your mobility at the neck and mid back.

- ▶ Your posture can influence the numbness and tingling felt along the arm.

You want to start with the neck, which means performing exercises 1 (gears) and 2 (cervical tucks). The basis of this prescription is that general mobility involving the neck, mid back, and low back can help the neurodynamics of your nerve, which in turn may help reduce the numbness and tingling down your arm. Exercise 3 (type 1 and 2 rotation) and foam rolling of your mid back will further enhance your nerve neurodynamics, thus reducing your current and future chance of discomfort and pain.

If your numbness and tingling become worse, immediately consult your physician. You don't want to do anything that aggravates the condition.

Ailment No. 3: Shoulder Pain

THE PROBLEM

When I was eighteen years old, I remember working out at a gym in Montreal and messing around with the pec deck machine. A sharp pain took over my right shoulder on my third rep, and I stopped and grasped it in agony. My shoulder wasn't the same after that, and I spent years trying to find a solution! Turns out, I'd experienced shoulder impingement because my excessive chest workouts were causing me to have a rounded back, and that ruined my shoulder mechanics.

DO THIS NOW: Stand up nice and tall and reach overhead with one arm. Pay attention to how this feels and how far you are able to reach. Now slouch forward and try this movement again. You'll find you can't reach as high as you did when you stood up straight.

Shoulder impingement and pain are common ailments affecting all age groups. A third of all people will deal with this discomfort in their lifetime. We all know someone who broke their shoulder from a fall because their dog saw a squirrel or dislocated their shoulder mountain biking because the jump didn't look that big ten seconds ago. But most shoulder pain isn't the result of trauma. It usually involves a combination of issues in the neck, trunk, and scapula. Though my exercises help with the mid back, it's important to note the importance of the scapula, otherwise known as the shoulder blade. There are four rotator cuff muscles that manifest from the scapula, and they attach to our arms to help stabilize the shoulder. These muscles need to be considered in performing any movements that require shoulder strength—for example, downward dog, TRX rows, or the rings in gymnastics. The scapular stabilizing muscles are important for your shoulders. I've provided an exercise that helps with scapular muscle awareness, strengthening, and neurological input to further enhance the postural exercises (Figure 8.3).

Once shoulder pain kicks in, it can be aggravated by specific movements and even sleep positions. Maybe your daily activities involve a lot of shoulder and overhead movements (shout-out to the painters, hairdressers, and others using their hands all day). Maybe you're just getting older. These are all things that can influence susceptibility to shoulder pain. This sort of pain rarely exists in isolation. Usually there are several culprits, including posture!

THE SOLUTION

Three principles can help simplify and guide your healing:

▶ You want the shoulder to move better.

▶ You want the shoulder to be stronger.

▶ You want the shoulder to be more stable.

Forcing a painful shoulder through its paces will only make things worse. Exercises 3 (type 1 and 2 rotation) and 4 (dynamic lat stretch) will help modify the thoracic spine posture and lengthen muscles that otherwise may be shortened in a painful shoulder. In addition, you want to foam roll the mid back for mobility. These movements will help your shoulder move better. And by addressing your posture and maximizing your shoulder mobility and strength, you can reduce shoulder pain and impingement, regardless of the conditions that may be present. Further, exercises 3 and 4 will provide a foundation that sets you up for success with the traditional shoulder exercises that are performed in Pilates and yoga studios as well as the gym! You can maximize traditional shoulder-strengthening exercises (e.g., the push-up) by enhancing your mid back and shoulder mobility.

Shoulders are finicky, and strengthening the stabilizing muscles of the shoulder and shoulder blades is key. Try this mobility and strength exercise to work on your shoulder stability:

1. Lie on your stomach with your arms behind your back, elbows up. Make a fist with both your hands and squeeze.

2. With your fisted hands facing down, straighten your arms so that they're off the floor. Maintain that squeeze.

3. With your arms off the floor, slowly bring them around behind your back while keeping them lifted. Maintain that hand squeeze. End in the T position. This should take a count of five seconds—don't rush the movement.

4. Reverse the movement back to the original start position.

5. An advanced version of this exercise is to end in a Y position, with your arms above your head as you lay flat on your stomach, both thumbs pointed up.

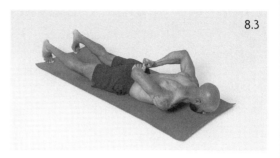

8.3

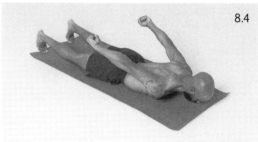

8.4

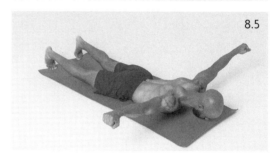

8.5

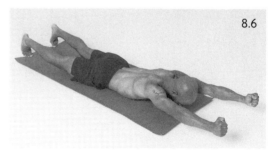

8.6

Continuous articular rotations for shoulder strength

Ailment No. 4: Disc Problems

THE PROBLEM

Disc problems mostly manifest as two conditions: disc bulges and arthritis. Among those aged thirty and above, disc bulges (and herniations) verge on being an epidemic in the United States and are twice as prevalent in men than women. Arthritis at the back (otherwise known as degenerative disc disease) is also increasing among those fifty and up, as shown in the thousands of X-rays performed every day. Together, disc bulges and arthritis make up most disc pathologies seen in orthopedics. Unfortunately, this has led to an abundance of fear. It's important to note that though the prevalence of disc pathologies has steadily increased, mobility and exercise *have* been shown to be effective in mitigating the negative effects of disc disease.

Susceptibility to disc problems is typically influenced by bad posture (e.g., hunching), bad movement habits (e.g., sitting too much), mechanical stress (e.g., lifting and bending forward for work), and weight gain. Muscle imbalances in the middle back and hips can play a big role.

However, it's important to note that up to 30 percent of disc herniations don't result in pain. So if you've had an MRI that reveals a disc herniation, that injury may or may not be associated with your lower back pain.

THE SOLUTION

People with disc problems often avoid doing particular movements for fear of doing further damage. If you can do an activity like bending forward without pain, don't be afraid to continue moving. I highly encourage movement!

▶ Disc problems are more common than you think, but they don't make it impossible to live your life.

▶ Mobility and exercise are key to reducing the consequences of disc problems.

Focusing on the variations of exercise 1 ("gears") can help with your general mobility from the head down to the toes. Doing exercises 5 (lateral bending) and 6 (McKenzie extension) can help address restrictions that may be present in disc herniation and degeneration. Exercise 5 helps alleviate low back disc pain by opening up the hips. Exercise 6 may help alleviate specific disc bulges in the lumbar spine. With both exercises, avoid any aggravation in the lower back. If it hurts, stop. I'll also point out that exercises 7 (3D psoas stretch), 9 (around the clock), and 10 (split stance hinge) can increase mobility that's been compromised by disc problems. Try using a foam roller, focusing on both sides of your glutes, quadriceps, hamstrings, and calf muscles. This can provide the appropriate stimulus to get your muscles moving.

Ailment No. 5: Sciatica

THE PROBLEM

Sciatica is pain radiating from the sciatic nerve down the lower back, hips, buttocks, and lower legs (Figure 8.7). It's typically felt on one side of the body. Sciatica is often diagnosed as a condition, but it should be noted that it's a symptom—meaning it's often the result of something else happening in the body. Sciatica is usually caused by disc pathologies in the lumbar spine or tightness in a hip muscle called the piriformis. Either can send pain shooting down the back of the leg. The sciatic nerve is the longest and thickest in the body. When the sciatic nerve is irritated, it can produce pain ranging from mild to severe, to the point of being debilitating. It can also produce numbness, tingling down the foot, and even muscle weakness in the leg and foot.

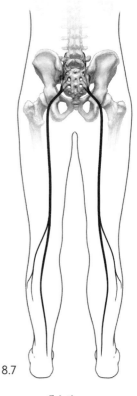

8.7

Sciatic nerve

Like the numbness and tingling down the arm that we previously discussed, sciatica is often associated with neurodynamics, meaning a lack of mobility of the sciatic nerve.

THE SOLUTION

Since sciatica often involves the sciatic nerve, and we've already learned that decreased neurodynamics can lead to sciatica, you want to do two things:

▸ Identify the position that aggravates your discomfort, and avoid prolonged exposure to this position (e.g., sitting).

▸ Focus on mobilizing the tissue that surrounds the sciatic nerve: the glute muscles, hamstring, and calf.

Because the sciatic nerve is present throughout the leg, exercises 5 (lateral bending), 6 (McKenzie extension), 7 (3D psoas stretch), 8 (hip stretch), 9 (around the clock), and 10 (split stance hinge) can help ease these symptoms. Any mobility work that doesn't aggravate your pain can reduce symptoms. Moreover, since tightness in the hips, buttocks, hamstrings, and calves can easily trap the sciatic nerve, mobilizing these muscles can help immensely. Try foam rolling your mid back and both sides of your glutes, hamstrings, and calf muscles.

Ailment No. 6: Tight Hips

If the front of your thighs or your butt muscles feels tight, your hips might be the culprit. Tight hips are usually the result of several shortened and tight muscles around the pelvis, resulting in pain or pinching in the front of the hips. Prolonged sitting will cause tightening of the hip flexors and the external rotators of the hips. The net effect of these muscles becoming tight is increased compression of the front of the hips. You may also notice this while you walk, taking shorter steps due to a "pulling sensation" felt at the front of your hips. You'll also feel it if you struggle to sit cross-legged as you did effortlessly in kindergarten. Even everyday activities, like sitting on a soft and low couch, can produce this feeling. Suddenly your tight hips can make everyday mundane movements annoying to deal with.

THE SOLUTION

Hip tightness can have multiple causes, but I believe it's often a sign that you're not moving sufficiently throughout your day. Integrating my mobility exercises regularly through your waking hours and simply getting up more may greatly improve your feelings of tightness. Here are some principles you'll want to consider:

▶ Tightness and stiffness in your hips may be a result of immobility, which can manifest due to prolonged posture (e.g., sitting).

▶ Tightness at the hips occurs in all three planes of movement (as mentioned in chapter 5). If you don't address restrictions in one plane, this may lead to compensation in the other.

When people think of tight hips, they only think in terms of how well their hips move forward and back. This primarily concerns the sagittal plane. But they often forget that it's important for the hip to be able to move side to side (frontal) and rotate in and out freely (transverse). This is why doing my mobility exercises is essential for your hip mobility. They address the hips from all angles, and all sides.

You need to move to mitigate these symptoms, and my mobility exercises can help.

Make sure you attempt exercises 5 (lateral bending), 7 (3D psoas stretch), 8 (hip stretch), 9 (around the clock), and 10 (split stance hinge). Importantly, you want to focus on foam rolling your glutes, hamstrings, and quadriceps.

Ailment No. 7: Runner's Knee

THE PROBLEM

This common injury occurs at the front of the kneecap, just below the pointed end. It's an overuse injury related to repetitive stress in activities that emphasize the hips, pelvis, and foot (basically every activity from Barre fitness to fencing). Despite the name, runner's knee is not limited to runners!

If runner's knee is present, it's most noticeable with walking, moving up and down stairs, and squatting (e.g., sitting down on a chair or the toilet). For some, the knee pain can be accompanied by varying levels of swelling, popping, and clicking. It's clinically known as patellofemoral pain syndrome and is seen in every practice in the world.

It's important to note that the knee is directed by two bosses: the hip and the foot. They both are constantly feeding information to the knee, for better or for worse. Because of this, the knee is greatly influenced by the quality of movement available from above and below.

THE SOLUTION

If you're experiencing this pain, stop doing the aggravating activity until symptoms have fully dissipated. For example, if you find yourself experiencing pain after walking for more than fifteen minutes, wait a couple of days for inflammation to decrease and attempt a shorter time or distance on your next walk. If this feels good, slowly add more time or distance as tolerated. The same applies to jumping and running activities. Use your response to an activity to guide your activity tolerance. If doing the activity doesn't produce pain, it's likely okay for the knee. Here are some principles to consider when dealing with runner's knee:

▸ It's often associated with repetitive stress on the leg.

▸ Temporarily stopping the aggravating activity will help alleviate the pain in the short term.

▶ Mobility and strengthening exercises for the hip, knee, and feet can alleviate the pain.

Though the source of knee pain is the knee, remember that the back, hips, and feet influence the load placed on the knee. Therefore, any tightness or weakness in those areas can influence knee pain. Exercises 5 (lateral bending) and 7 (3D psoas stretch) help with hip mobility and load. Exercise 9 (around the clock), and 11 (foot pronation and supination) will allow you to maximize your range of motion and strength at the knees and feet. Finally, foam rolling your quadriceps, front shin, and calf muscles can greatly alleviate discomfort. If the problem persists, see a physical therapist or physician for further investigation. Otherwise, you want to futureproof your knees by doing these exercises.

Ailment No. 8: Plantar Fasciitis

THE PROBLEM

Plantar fasciitis is inflammation of the plantar fascia fibrous tissue that supports the bottom of the feet and gives them an arch. Usually the tissue grows irritated from poor foot mobility and walking mechanics. A stiff foot will lead to an inflexible plantar fascia, which in turn will cause uneven distribution of pressure when you walk.

In a normal gait, different parts of the foot need to move in opposite directions to produce efficient motion (it's similar to how your torso and pelvis move in opposition to each other while walking). When there is no opposition going on in a stiff foot, the plantar fascia can't stretch and contract the way it needs to, and pressure accumulates at one spot. You end up with pain and inflammation.

Plantar fasciitis—as well as other foot problems, for that matter—is often prevalent in those who have gained weight, especially if the weight gain happened relatively quickly (i.e., a 5 to 20 percent increase in weight in less than a year). The increased load can influence foot mechanics, altering how your foot moves.

THE SOLUTION

Currently, the most common solution is introducing an orthotic, that thing you put in your shoe. Orthotics can serve as a Band-Aid, but eventually, you'll need to live without them. You should focus on developing mobility and strength of the foot without any aid. Therefore, all the exercises I recommend should be done barefoot. These are the main concepts you want to consider:

▶ Plantar fasciitis often results from a change in load on the foot, and is typically influenced by repetitive stressors like overuse or weight gain.

▶ Orthotics can be helpful but are considered a Band-Aid solution.

▶ Focusing on mobility and strength of the foot is key.

Adopting proper foot mechanics and strengthening exercises are essential. To improve your foot mobility, I would focus on exercises 11 (foot pronation and supination) and 12 (big toe extension). Foam rolling your front shin and calf muscles can influence the tension onto your foot and may temporarily help alleviate some of the symptoms of plantar fasciitis. I'd also recommend easing off on any activity that worsens the pain and wearing footwear that doesn't exacerbate it. However, it's important to remember that the long-term solution must involve exercising your feet.

Ailment No. 9: Shin Splints

THE PROBLEM

This is typically an overuse injury caused by some combination of running and walking more than usual, an increase in the speed of foot pronation (arch lowering) in the walking cycle, and tight calf muscles. Naturally, it's best to work on exercises for control of the hips and strengthening the calf and foot. Shin splints don't exist in isolation, being a manifestation of how you walk and run. If your core is weak, your hip mobility is poor along multiple planes of movement, and your running isn't efficient, your susceptibility to shin splints will greatly increase.

Shin splints must be differentiated from stress fractures. Stress fractures are cracks in your bone; shin splints are inflammation in muscles, tendons, and bone around the tibia. Both conditions arise from an overload issue and originate below the knee. How can you tell if you have a stress fracture versus a shin splint?

▶ Stress fractures present at a local region along the shin and will get worse with an activity like running.

▶ Shin splints tend to be broad along the shin, and the pain tends to decrease if you mobilize and warm up before your activity—for example, foam roll and perform active movements of the ankle before running.

To be on the safe side, it's best to consult a healthcare professional (ideally, a physician) to ensure you're not dealing with a fracture. This will usually require an X-ray, a bone scan, or an MRI.

THE SOLUTION

Similar to the management of plantar fasciitis, shin splints require that you pay attention to the activity that may be contributing to the pain and find exercises that can help you get back to your goals of walking, jogging, running, and every activity associated with these movements. There are a couple of principles you want to consider:

▶ Make sure that what you're dealing with is shin splints and not a stress fracture of the bone. Either way, it's best to identify the activity that may be causing pain (e.g., running) and resting from it. Once the pain improves, you want to gradually reintroduce the original activity that led to your discomfort (e.g., walk briskly pain-free before trying a light jog or run).

▶ Mobility of the hip, knee, and foot is key to addressing shin splints.

For the hips, you'll want to focus on exercises 5 (lateral bending), 7 (3D psoas stretch), 8 (hip stretch), 9 (around the clock), and 10 (split stance hinge). To optimize foot mechanics, you'll want to do exercises 11 (foot pronation and supination) and 12 (big toe extension). Foam roll your calf muscles and shins to address muscular imbalances and trigger points.

Ailment No. 10: Low Back Pain

THE PROBLEM

Low back pain is the most common injury I've seen—and it's the most debilitating injury economically. Nearly 80 percent of people in America will experience low back pain. The cost of this is estimated at $100 billion a year.

What makes low back pain so complicated is that there are so many conditions that may contribute to it: disc bulges, arthritis, ligament damage, pregnancy, muscular strain, muscle imbalance, hip mechanics, knee mechanics, foot mechanics, and everything in between. It might hurt when you sit, it might hurt when you stand, or it might hurt only when you try too advanced a pose in yoga class or lift too heavy in the gym. Regardless, low back pain is multifactorial and complex in its diagnosis.

With any back pain you notice, it's important for you to know a few important things:

▸ If you're experiencing loss of function of your bowel or bladder, you want to consult a doctor immediately.

▸ If you've recently been immobilized for a period of time (e.g., postpartum), you may experience protracted low back pain.

▸ Low back pain can be acute (e.g., from a recent sudden injury) or chronic (involving a gradual buildup of pain over time).

▶ There's a strong argument for increasing mobility in addressing low back pain, regardless of cause.

Low back pain may be the most common condition I see with my clients, but thankfully I have an arsenal of mobility tools to combat it. And the most common exercises I use have been provided in this book.

THE SOLUTION

A simple way to think about low back pain is this: Look above and below the area of pain. If your low back hurts, odds are you have a stiff hip joint (below) or a stiff thoracic spine (above). Your low back is probably compensating for the lack of movement and strength in these other areas.

Mobility is key to addressing low back pain, since it can both serve as a test for your movement capacity and alleviate devious symptoms. If what is influencing the lower back pain is coming from above the waist, you'll want to focus on exercises 3 (type 1 and 2 rotation), 4 (dynamic lat stretch), and 6 (McKenzie extension). If the influence on the back pain is from the waist down, you'll want to focus on exercises 5 (lateral bending), 7 (3D psoas stretch), 8 (hip stretch), 9 (around the clock), 10 (split stance hinge), and 11 (foot pronation and supination). To focus on trigger points that may be related to low back pain, use a foam roller for your mid back, glutes, quadriceps, hamstrings, and calf muscles.

If the list above looks exhaustive, it's because there's a theme that I'm highlighting. Whether the root problem is occurring above the low back or below it, addressing low back pain boils down to focusing on exercises for the thoracic spine, hip mobility, knee mobility, and foot mobility.

To Perform Better, Recover Better

Recovery often refers to coming back from an illness or injury. Another definition of recovery is a set of activities (e.g., mobility stretches, manual therapy, ice, heat) tacked on to the end of a workout. But the third form of recovery is the time between someone's training and when their physical and mental function returns to its pre-workout baseline. Whether the event is a marathon or Olympic lifting, recovery is complete only when the body returns to the state it was in before the marathon or the workout. The duration of this recovery period is based on all sorts of variables. For instance, after a marathon, it might take the casual endurance athlete a week to recover fully, but a world-class marathoner will likely return to baseline a few days after their event.

Recovery can be lengthened or shortened depending on a person's actions. For example, after a grueling workout at the gym, the following night's sleep always affects recovery. Eight hours of deep sleep will enhance it; three hours of fitful sleep will impair it.

Concerning mobility, recovery requires reestablishing your baseline range of motion and your baseline strength to ensure you can participate in the activities you wish to pursue. Suppose you're a runner who has sustained an injury or has become exhausted from a challenging run. In that case, recovering your mobility means running again at the same capacity. You can use my exercises to get a sense of your overall mobility, ensuring you can return to your desired sport and futureproofing your body for anything.

9

THE CHALLENGES FACING SPECIFIC GROUPS

BESIDES OFFERING SPECIFIC prescriptions for the ten common health ailments, we also need to pay special attention to the needs of particular populations. These are not small subsets of people: I'm talking about women and men, older people, runners, people who drive a lot, and athletes playing particular sports. These groups are often prone to specific problems. For example, shin splints are a classic runner's injury.

I could write an entire book about the mobility regimen that might be appropriate for someone with osteoarthritis or Parkinson's disease. Of course, those are complex disease processes, and every patient is different. Any physical therapy advice I'd give such a patient would be highly individualized. If you have any questions about the content of this book as it applies to your specific condition, consult with your doctor. Typically, specific medical conditions have contraindications to them—e.g., if you've had a recent heart attack, you can't participate in physical or cardiovascular activity until you've been cleared by a physician. That said, when a serious illness is present (e.g., Parkinson's), mobility exercises done safely are almost always recommended in the literature. Bed rest is rarely a recipe for longevity.

Listen to your body, though. If you have a chronic pain condition like fibromyalgia, you're probably used to seeing how your body responds when you attempt an activity. If it's painful or uncomfortable, you should back off—you've already been down that road. Sometimes you can't do certain things at certain times. I'm not a fan of gutting through an activity thinking, *I'm in agonizing pain, but I'll keep doing it. Then I'll feel better.* It seldom works that way, I'm afraid. Try cutting back on your intensity a little bit until you find the level your body can tolerate. No one but you can say what that level is.

If You're Older . . .

To state the obvious: a typical eighty-year-old does not have the posture or the mobility of a twenty-year-old. Young people have had fewer injuries and less time for bad habits to develop. Their movement patterns tend to be much cleaner and more efficient. But over time, injuries and bad habits can begin piling up. The resulting poor mechanics grind away at joints, irritating muscles that are asked to do more than they were designed for.

The aging process also involves natural forces that inevitably take a toll. For example, gravity can significantly affect our posture and influence the load placed on the body. Erik Dalton, PhD, a manual therapist, educator, and author, talks about the never-ending battle between gravity and a person's strength, with posture being a scorecard as to which side is winning and losing. At a certain point, your body is no longer the constant ally it once was. It's less forgiving. There are visible changes; for example, the average person's skeleton shrinks half an inch or so per decade. The loss is even greater after seventy. The discs between the spine's vertebrae no longer provide as much cushion or space as they once did. The skeleton also tends to begin leaning forward, further diminishing a person's stature. Gravity gradually gains the upper hand.

BONE LOSS

Losses in bone density, strength, and mass accelerate with age. NASA has extensively researched the changes the human body goes through while in space, and bone loss may be the most significant of them all, if only because bone is the most challenging part of the body to recoup. Astronauts lose up to 1 percent per month of their bone mineral density in space, most significantly in their lower back, pelvis, and hips. The human body is smart. Bones aren't stressed in the absence of gravity, so the body doesn't send them calcium in space. Bones start releasing calcium. This bone loss becomes apparent in astronauts' urine when they're tested. So when astronauts return to Earth after a mission, NASA makes sure they're taking a multivitamin, getting enough calcium, drinking enough milk—basic stuff. It's not rocket science. (Sorry, I had to say that once.)

NASA also has to figure out ways to load the body in the weightless environment of space. If a 150-pound astronaut can squat 250 pounds on Earth, 350 pounds of load somehow must be applied in the weightlessness of space. Scientists devote a lot of time and energy to figuring out the best exercise countermeasures to minimize the losses of the bone, muscle, and cardiovascular tissues so humans can go to Mars and beyond one day.

Here on Earth, inactivity leads to bone loss. The process is gradual and more closely tied to aging. When the spine loses bone, it leads to greater curvature and even more forward lean. What's more, the collagen that helps form bones, tendons, and other connective tissues grows less elastic and more brittle. Medications like steroids, diuretics, and opioids can lessen bone density. Habits like smoking and excessive alcohol consumption are also detrimental to our bones and connective tissue.

Little wonder, then, that bone fractures imperil the elderly. These fractures typically stem from a condition called osteoporosis, which is the weakening of the bones through decreased bone mass, verified through bone density scans. It is estimated that there are 200 million people in the world with hip fractures associated with osteoporosis. Osteoporosis afflicts both sexes but particularly women. And as women age, the prevalence of osteoporosis increases significantly with each decade. These fractures tend to strike the hips, spine, and forearms. Unfortunately, these fractures tend to be a result of falls. Alarmingly, falls are the leading cause of injury-related death among adults sixty-five and older, and the mortality rate from a fall increases as we age.

A frail human body becomes vulnerable to external forces that younger, healthier bodies shrug off. When young people trip and stub their toe, they recover their balance and go on about their business, the only fallout being a slight embarrassment. As the elderly lose strength, muscle, bone density, coordination, and balance, the smallest trigger can set a fall in motion. Because elderly bones are brittle, they break in response to less and less impact. The hip bones are the most common part of the skeleton to fracture in a fall. In fact, among those fifty and older, falls account for nearly 300,000 hip fractures per year in the United States. Many of these falls are a result of environmental factors (e.g., poor lighting, tripping obstacles, and slippery surfaces). Thankfully, we've seen that physical therapy intervention can reduce falls in the elderly by up to 30 percent.

Is there a way to reduce the risk of falling? First, ensure that the environment in which you live has as few hazards as possible (e.g., proper lighting and no clutter on the floor—and don't forget to get your eyes checked!). Second, you need to exercise. This includes walking, climbing the stairs, basic sit-to-stand progressions, and my exercises that focus on the hips and legs. With any exercise you participate in, you want to make sure that the environment is safe and that you have something to hold on to.

MUSCLE LOSS

We produce less testosterone and growth hormone, critical catalysts for muscle growth, starting around age thirty. After that age, the body also begins steadily losing muscle mass every year, amounting to a loss of 5 to 10 percent between twenty-four and fifty. Less muscle means less support for the spine and more posture problems. Along with the back muscles, the glutes and hamstrings play a critical role in spine health. Many back injuries result from tight or weak glutes and hamstrings that force people into awkward positions. All the mobility exercises I have offered for the lower body will help your spine stay in good condition.

I'm sure you can see a trend here. Various forces work to cause the body to lean forward and to make bones more brittle. When you see an older person hunched over and shuffling along, most likely all of these factors are at work.

As alarming as that sounds, there's more. Many, if not all, physiological and bio-mechanical parameters measuring fitness and wellness naturally worsen as we age. Metabolism, endurance, flexibility, and bone mineral density peak between ages twenty-five to thirty, then slowly and steadily decline. Strength peaks at roughly twenty-five, plateaus through thirty-five to forty, and then drops at an accelerating pace, with a 25 percent loss of peak force by age sixty-five.

The good news is that the changes brought on by aging *are* incremental, and they can be minimized and managed by following my plan. Often the physical decline among those who are older relates less to the aging process than to the lifestyle changes accompanying it. For example, while your metabolism holds fairly constant until age sixty, decreasing the amount of exercise you get *will* set in motion a cascade of negative physical effects.

If you're sixty-five years or older, you need to focus on your mobility. Once you have that as your foundation, start working on control and focusing on the daily activities that are important to you—e.g., sit-to-stand exercises to strengthen the legs so that you can sit on a chair without collapsing. Finally, focusing on strength and stability is of prime importance because it's the most straightforward thing you can alter in an aging body.

If You're a Woman . . .

People often ask me whether the posture hygiene routine that works for men works equally well for women and vice versa. When it comes to physical fitness, the sexes are more similar than different. Often the differences that *are* highlighted or accentuated are more for marketing purposes than anything meaningful. A good example is the dietary supplement industry. There's an adage that when a company wants to market a supplement line for women, they "shrink it and pink it": that is, they take essentially the same product, make it a smaller size, and package it in pink. Voilà, a product made for women.

Most programs that work well for men will work well for women, too, including this one. That's not to say there aren't differences between the sexes; it's just that the differences tend to be superficial. Men naturally carry more muscle than women, but that doesn't mean that foam rolling the kinks in that muscle tissue isn't equally important. Men and women have different arrays of hormones, too. Men naturally have much more testosterone, helping them build and support more muscle. But again, your sex shouldn't make much difference in terms of this program or any other.

I've noticed in my clinics that women are more prone than men to neck and shoulder symptoms, and there's some research supporting this anecdotal observation. Women are twice as likely as men to suffer neck and shoulder issues related to using touchscreen devices. We've already established that a chronically rounded back leads to all manner of health issues, but here's the kicker: The thoracic spine will start rounding simply from the aging process, starting as early as in your mid-twenties. This tendency of the back to round with aging accelerates even faster in women than men. Rounding is terrible for mobility, predisposing older women to degenerative disc disease, osteoporosis, and compression fractures of the thoracic spine.

Along with neck pain, low back pain is the most common complaint I hear from patients. Women are even more likely than men to experience low back pain, a difference that starts in elementary school and continues through old age. Women also tend to live longer than men. You can see the issue: Not only are women more prone to back injuries, they're also living longer with those injuries.

THE PELVIC FLOOR

In 2013, a strange situation began sparking comment in the CrossFit universe. Because of how hard the CrossFit workouts were, many participants, particularly women, were literally peeing during heavy lifts. It became such a common occurrence that people started considering it normal. Well, it may be common (it has been reported that up to 90 percent of women who experience low back pain experience pelvic floor dysfunction), but that doesn't mean we should accept it. I'm no expert in pelvic floor health, but I do know that this dysfunction takes the following forms:

▶ Incontinence—that is, bladder and bowel leakage while you do an activity (like exercise), when you cough/sneeze, or when you really have an urge to urinate or have a bowel movement but can't control yourself sufficiently to make it on time.

▶ Pelvic organ prolapse—that is, a bulge and drooping of your uterus, bladder, or rectum due to muscle weakness.

▶ Difficulty emptying your bowel or bladder completely, and the pain associated with this.

I recommend that if you do experience any of the above symptoms (even the slightest), you seek the guidance of a primary healthcare practitioner. That said, at Myodetox we now have several therapists who specialize in pelvic health, and increasingly, women and men are coming to us to seek help with this significant issue.

Exercise Guidelines If You're Pregnant or Postpartum

For the pregnant and postpartum women reading my book, I want you to know that my exercises are generally safe and beneficial for you. But before you participate in them, please follow the guidelines below.

Pregnancy

▷ Pregnant women should seek medical clearance from their doctor for physical activity as they progress through pregnancy.

▷ All women cleared by their physician for exercise should be physically active throughout their pregnancy.

▷ Pregnant women should try to accumulate at least 150 minutes of moderate-intensity physical activity, including cardiovascular exercise (for example, walking), mobility (e.g., all the exercises in chapter 6), and strength training (e.g., squats, exercises in chapter 6). This should be done three days a week at a minimum, more if possible.

▷ Pregnant women should train their pelvic floor muscles, which is best prescribed by a physiotherapist or other health practitioners who specialize in the pelvic floor.

▷ Pregnant women should avoid exercise if they experience light-headedness, nausea, or any feelings of uneasiness.

Postpartum

▷ Postpartum women should seek medical clearance from their physician before attempting physical activity.

▷ The same principles apply to postpartum women as to pregnant women.

Posture and Your Bag

Many factors can throw off your posture and negatively affect your mobility over the course of a day. One, for example, is carrying a weighted bag on your shoulder, whether you're a student lugging a laptop carrying case or a mom carrying a diaper bag. There's a temptation to put all sorts of things into a bag: electronic devices, gym clothes, makeup—you name it. Unfortunately, creating an unbalanced load on one shoulder can force the body into unnatural adjustments (Figure 9.1). What's more, the muscles up around the base of the neck, called the upper trapezius, often seize up, eventually leading to neck pain and other problems.

Relatively simple strategies can mitigate the damage. First, don't take quite as much stuff with you; leave behind what's nonessential. Second, find a bag with a long enough strap that you can sling the bag across your body. So if the strap is slung over your right shoulder, the bag should hang on your left side. That way, the pressure is more evenly distributed on both sides. It's not perfect, but it's better than having the strap on one shoulder and the bag hanging straight down, yanking your body in that direction.

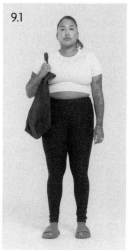 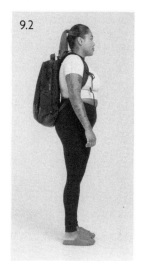

9.1   9.2

Uneven distribution   *Even distribution*

Another thing to consider is a backpack (Figure 9.2). When you put one on your back, the weight is more evenly distributed than with the strap on one shoulder and the bag on the other side. It's easier to carry, too. Maybe it doesn't make the best fashion statement, but there are some pretty cool-looking backpacks out there nowadays.

LUMBAR LORDOSIS

Lordosis refers to excessive inward curving of the lumbar spine. Women tend to have more significant lumbar lordosis than men, which may be related to childbirth and rearing. This increased curvature at the lumbar spine for women may serve an essential purpose—namely, reducing the load on the back during pregnancy. But this comes with consequences like decreased lumbar spine stability, decreased core strength, and increased pain. Conversely, those with "flat back" are more likely to experience increased risk of disc problems.

In my clinics I see more posterior pelvic tilt among men and more anterior pelvic tilt among women. The direction of these tilts may have some influence on lower back pain. Posterior pelvic tilt leads to more rounding of the lower back, which unfortunately increases the risk of injury to the lumbar spine discs.

With anterior tilt, there tends to be more compression of low back structures and tightened back muscles. This is most associated with lumbar lordosis and is common among my pregnant patients. Like we discussed earlier, the weight of a developing fetus shifts a woman's center of mass forward, leading to an increase in lordosis and an anterior pelvic tilt. Therefore, the risk of low back pain increases as women progress through their pregnancy.

Though it's beyond the scope of this book, if you have a posterior pelvic tilt, you'll want to focus on lumbar mobility. If you have an anterior pelvic tilt, you'll want to work on core strength.

GENDER DIFFERENCES IN MUSCLE

Hamstring tightness is associated with lower back pain, and there's some speculation that during resistance training, women have a harder time than men activating their hamstring muscles. It's an unresolved debate, but there could be something there.

The gluteus maximus and gluteus medius muscles (the butt, in simple terms) also help explain why low back pain affects women more than it does men. The glutes help stabilize the pelvis, and weak glutes tend to be correlated with low back pain. Weakness of the gluteus medius is more common in women than men. This weakness is present because in general women have a wider pelvis than men, and this greater width stresses the gluteus medius more.

Women are sometimes said to have more issues with pelvic pain than men, and statistically that's true—but not to the degree many people think. One difference, of course, is that some women go through childbirth, which might require strengthening or otherwise working on the pelvic floor more than men. Relaxin, a hormone released naturally, especially during pregnancy, creates more lax ligaments and may contribute to increased low back and pelvic pain. All the more important to ensure you have a well-balanced pelvis with a full range of motion and optimal strength to decrease the adverse effects of any hormonal changes.

That's not to say men don't need to do pelvic work; they do. One thing that helps perpetuate stereotypes is that men are taught not to discuss pelvic issues, to just grin and bear it. But as I mentioned earlier, pelvic floor dysfunction can also occur in men.

If You're a Runner . . .

It's estimated that 36 million people run in the United States, and nearly 80 percent will report an injury to a lower extremity in their lifetime. I want you to move more and sit less, so it may surprise you to hear me say anything negative about running. After all, it's one way to move. But because running is so complex biomechanically, be mindful of certain realities.

For starters, running places a much greater load on the body than standing still or walking. When you stand, two strong pillars, your legs, support your body weight. When you walk, you always have at least one foot on the ground for support. But when you run, you're technically falling forward, and there are moments in the run cycle where both feet are off the ground. That dramatically increases the stress applied to your bones, tendons, muscles, and ligaments every time one of your feet makes contact. As a result, running will lay bare any issues you have with posture, biomechanics, flexibility, mobility, balance, and stability. In such cases, your knees and ankles are particularly vulnerable to injury.

If you're a runner, my posture hygiene regimen should help immensely. I'm not saying to avoid running—just to be careful and mix it up with other forms of cardio. If the goal is to elevate your heart rate, you can achieve the same effect by doing a stationary bike class or walking on a treadmill set at an incline, neither of which should negatively affect your knees.

One way to decrease the force running places on the joints is to shorten your stride, leading to more frequent steps. Serious runners refer to this step rate as cadence, or steps per minute. The ideal cadence is around 180 steps per minute, regardless of the speed you're running. You can figure out your steps per minute on a treadmill or with your smart watch by counting the number of times you strike your left (or right) foot on the ground in a minute and multiplying that by two. Injury risk tends to increase if your cadence is less than 180.

Adjusting your cadence is best done on a treadmill because it's a more controlled environment than outdoors. You can maintain the same pace on a treadmill and quickly notice how changing a single variable (stride/cadence) affects your running form. Your running posture should become more relaxed, with much less shock absorption through your low back, hips, and knees.

When it comes to progressing your running, you should always increase your distance gradually, no more than 10 percent a week. So if you run five miles one week, don't run more than five and a half miles the following week. Moreover, you should be running at a pace in which you're able to talk while you run. Why? Because the ability to talk indicates that you're in control of your breathing, and that you're not straining your breathing and heart to the point of excessive exertion.

Running Posture

Let's try a home experiment. I want you to stand tall, with your trunk and knees straight. Now lean forward. You'll find yourself naturally wanting to catch yourself with one foot to avoid falling. This is called "falling forward." Now assume a half-squat position with your knees bent and your trunk bent. Now when you lean forward, you'll notice that you're not falling forward. Your muscles are working hard to control this position. But do you want your muscles working this hard as you run? You'll end up putting more stress on your body if you do so. This is the "bent forward" position and uses more energy, making your muscles work hard and increasing your risk for injury (Figure 9.3). "Falling forward" is the better technique (Figure 9.4), one that puts less stress on your body as you run.

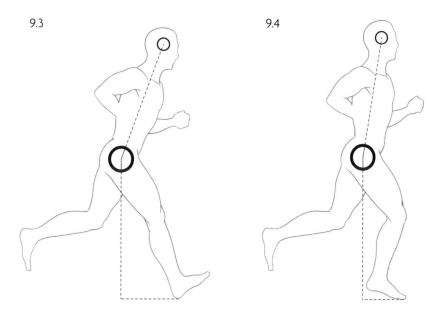

9.3

9.4

Trunk flexed, "bent forward"　　　　　*Upright, "falling forward"*

What exercises from this book should you do for running? Well, since the activity involves the trunk, back, hips, knees, and ankles, I suggest you do exercises 5 (lateral bending), 7 (3D psoas stretch), 8 (hip stretch), 9 (around the clock), 10 (split stance hinge), 11 (foot pronation and supination), and 12 (big toe extension). Finally, before and after runs, regularly use a foam roller in the following regions: your mid back, stomach, glutes, hamstrings, calf muscles, quadriceps, and shins.

If You Drive a Lot . . .

Driving can be a landmine for good posture. One leg is extended for long periods, putting excessive tension into the posterior chain, sciatic nerve, and pelvis. Many people spend hours a day behind the wheel, particularly in the new age of the gig economy. Those trapped in metropolitan commutes can spend a couple of hours or more in the car every day. Work-from-home policies have relieved many of this daily torment, but when people need to commute to the office, the spines of many commuters will pay the price.

Many of us sit awkwardly when we drive. Often we'll place one hand on top of the wheel and shift our torso in the opposite direction. Instead of the spine's aligning straight up and down, as it's supposed to, it moves into a configuration that resembles either an S shape or reverse S shape—the exact misalignment seen in scoliosis patients. The lack of mindfulness about how we're seated can have consequences. Often we'll exit the car and continue to favor one side or the other depending on how we were sitting.

"Hey," you might say, "I need to get around. Who can pay attention to this stuff?" *You* can if you decide it's important. Here's how to sit in a way that limits the stress on the spine. Try and maintain an upright, alert posture. Ideally, the seat back shouldn't be at 90 degrees; it should be tilted back a little, so the angle is more like 100 or 110 degrees. The top of the headrest should be between the top of your head and the tips of your ears. Your lumbar spine should lightly touch the seat. Ideally, your hips should be slightly higher than your knees, with a bit of space between the seat and your legs. Your line of sight should be at least three inches above the top of the steering wheel, and you should be able to grasp the wheel comfortably with a slight bend in the elbows. Position the mirrors so you can see comfortably without craning your neck.

Road trips have become a popular pastime during the pandemic when alternatives like flying and taking cruises haven't been available. On extended drives, use the techniques outlined above. If possible, take a break every hour or so, pulling off the road to a safe spot, well away from traffic. Various stretches I've discussed work well here and can be done standing during your stops. I would most recommend exercises 1 (gears), 2 (cervical tuck), and 3 (type 1 and 2 rotation). When you get back in your vehicle, it may have a button that returns you to your former ideal sitting position. If you need to change it for some reason, like to let a kid into the back seat, you can just push the button and your former seat position will be reestablished. If there's no button, manually make sure that your seat is in the proper place and that your mirrors are correctly positioned. This attention to detail will help you maintain good spine health and posture, enabling you to get safely and comfortably to where you want to go.

If You Play Sports . . .

BOXING

The Problem

In a boxing stance, your thoracic cage and pelvis are always coiled like a spring, readying the body to throw a punch. Meanwhile, your neck is constantly rotated while your gaze locks in on the target. This constant rotation can irritate the joints, muscles, and nerves in that region.

Sadly, rotator cuff impingement is very common among those who box. The constant twisting of the shoulder into internal rotation adds to the crazy concentric and eccentric forces traveling through the shoulder when throwing a punch. Pull one of your arms across your body. Feel a pinch in your shoulder? If so, you've likely developed some degree of shoulder impingement.

The Solution

One muscle that exerts a ton of eccentric load is the lats—especially when you throw a punch and miss. Keep this muscle mobile to prevent pinching of those rotator cuff structures. Foam rolling your lats while lying on your side with an arm overhead is the most efficient way. Spend time improving rotational mobility in the opposite direction. When you rotate to the opposite side you'll notice where you're tight and where you're over-lengthened. Keep your neck and shoulder mobile. Your key exercises will be 1 (gears), 2 (cervical tuck), 3 (type 1 and 2 rotation), and 4 (dynamic lat stretch) to set you up to throw an optimal punch.

GOLF

The Problem

Golf, like boxing, requires you to wind up your body like a slingshot. Unleashing the swing at a high level requires excellent hip rotation. People who have tight hips will have difficulty achieving maximal windup and follow-through. In straining to generate maximum power, they'll put immediate stress on the low back.

Sit in a chair and bring a knee as close as possible to your chest. Try and pull your knee toward the opposite shoulder from that position while keeping the knee fully bent. If you feel a pinch, you lack rotation in your hips and are likely irritating the structures in your hip.

The Solution

The main focus for golf is boosting the rotational mobility of the thoracic spine, shoulder, and hips by doing exercises 1 (all gears variations), 3 (type 1 and 2 rotation), and 10 (split stance hinge). Second, you want to optimize the mobility in your feet, since this can maximize the mobility achieved by your shoulder, mid back, and hips as you swing. Add exercise 11 (foot pronation and supination) as a way to train your foot to master your swing. In fact, golf's rotational aspects can be applied to all sports involving throwing and swinging: tennis, football, baseball, and everything in between.

MULTIDIRECTIONAL SPORTS
(E.G., SOCCER, FOOTBALL, BASKETBALL)

The Problem

Multidirectional sports place a high degree of stress on the pelvis and low back. Changing directions at various speeds, acceleration, and deceleration require a certain level of core control coupled with upper and lower extremity strength. When we lack this control but continue to pursue these sports, the most common strategy is to brace with the next best thing, usually the hip flexors, adductors (groin), and hip rotators.

Lie on your back. Cross your right foot over your left knee. Feel a pinch in your right hip and or butt cheek? Feel a pull in your right groin? Answer yes to any of these questions, and you've begun clenching your hip girdle muscles, likely to compensate for issues elsewhere.

The Solution

Spend time foam rolling out the adductors and hip rotators. Developing core strength will help prevent injuries when you lunge, pivot, and stop and start on the playing field or court. To maximize your mobility, you'll want to spend time on exercises 3 (type 1 and 2 rotation), 7 (3D psoas stretch), 8 (hip stretch), and 9 (around the clock).

CYCLING

The Problem

Cycling is one of the world's most popular activities, second only to running. Its popularity has soared in the form of stationary bike classes, whether at home or in a studio setting. But while cycling does a great job working the heart, lungs, and legs, it would be misleading not to point out the obvious: cycling often involves sitting at an extreme angle for prolonged periods. Therefore, fans of two-wheeled propulsion prepare yourself: In pursuing your favorite activity, you'll be susceptible to the same issues confronted by those who sit typing at a keyboard for hours or who spend long periods in the driver's seat.

The Solution

Exercises that encourage the opposite of all these prolonged postures are essential. Because cycling involves sitting, the list is long and necessary. These include all variations of exercises 1 (gears), 2 (cervical tuck), 3 (type 1 and 2 rotation), 5 (lateral bending), 7 (3D psoas stretch), 8 (hip mobility), 9 (around the clock), and 10 (split stance hinge and reach). The goal is to extend your thoracic spine, open up your chest, and stretch out your hip flexors. Don't neglect stretching your hamstrings, which are used even more if you're clipped to your bike. Lastly, you'll want to make sure that you're foam rolling your mid back, stomach, glutes, quadriceps, hamstrings, calf muscles, and shin muscles.

If you're participating in a traditional strength-training program for cycling, glute strength also needs developing. These muscles hardly get used during cycling because their primary function is lateral stabilization of the pelvis. The bike's frame artificially creates lateral stability, so on a bike these muscles never get the call. You'll want to make sure that overall, the strength exercises you work on emphasize what's *not* as utilized in cycling.

SWIMMING

The Problem

Swimming is an amazing whole-body workout that promotes both strength and cardiovascular fitness. However, swimmers often have problems with their shoulders—rotator cuff impingement is termed "swimmer's shoulder" for a reason. Many people with rotator cuff impingement have compromised shoulder mobility, but swimmers tend to have excessive mobility.

Being in the water is also somewhat unnatural because gravity doesn't exert the same force. So your body is playing in a new environment and following a different set of rules. It would make sense that a body efficient in an altered state of gravity would potentially be inefficient under the normal confines of gravity.

With your right hand, reach over your right shoulder as if you're scratching your back. Simultaneously, reach under and up with your left hand. The goal is to try to bring your hands together. Repeat with the opposite side. If your hands can't touch or you feel discomfort in either shoulder, you lack adequate shoulder mobility.

The Solution

In chapter 8, I went into detail about managing and mitigating shoulder impingement. For swimmers, the same principles apply:

- ► You want the shoulder to move better.

- ► You want the shoulder to be strong.

- ► You want the shoulder to be stable.

Exercises 3 (type 1 and 2 rotation) and 4 (dynamic lat stretch) will optimize your mid back and shoulder mobility as you focus on swimming. In addition, you want to foam roll the mid back. These will help your shoulder move better. Don't forget the highlighted exercises in chapter 8 (Figure 8.3) for shoulder impingement. The T and Y movement exercises allow swimmers to both identify and strengthen the shoulder in areas of compromised range of movement.

10 YOUR SPINE DOESN'T OPERATE IN A VACUUM

THE QUESTION BECOMES, "How can I integrate this into my lifestyle?" Whether you come to this book as someone completely inexperienced with mobility or as an avid participant in an activity, it's important to start following my posture and mobility hygiene plan. Futureproofing your spine and participating in the activities you want to do can only benefit and maximize your body's potential. Ignoring your posture and neglecting the body's mobility will result in poor outcomes, whether you live at the gym or sit on the couch all day. To make sure you fully absorb the key principles, let's revisit the 3 C's: creation, control, and capacity.

Control—Your Body and Your Core

Much of my book has focused on creation, control, and capacity, as discussed extensively in chapter 5. Arguably, many of the Big Twelve exercises and their variations focus on *creation* of space through mobility movements. Each one contains an aspect of *control*, in that baseline strength is required to do them well. *Capacity* develops when you do my exercises repetitively with ease, and when you start seeing postural changes in your everyday life. But one aspect that hasn't been touched on is core control.

Core control is essential for both static and dynamic (moving) posture. Core exercises include crunches, sit-ups, and planks, with an eye toward six-packs and strong obliques. But your core is so much more than just a flat, hard stomach. It's the area of your body through which all the force you bring to bear is transmitted. It involves muscles that surround your trunk and pelvic floor, and it enables strength, stability, and efficiency in movement. Core control is about creating rigidity for specific activities (such as lifting or carrying) or explosive power (such as with throwing or kicking). What's crucial in performing these activities is that the pelvic girdle and torso be stable relative to the arms and legs.

You must be able to maintain some stability while moving. When there's a disconnect between the two, bad things can happen. A perfect example is someone who has developed tight hip flexors (e.g., a hockey player, gymnast, or dancer). Such a person will be pulled into an anterior pelvic tilt in almost all their activities. Now imagine this same person decides to take up running. As they launch themselves in the air, they cannot fully disassociate and extend their hip from the lower back; as a result, they put an incredible amount of stress on the lower back. They've replaced their core with their tight hip flexors (and likely, the external rotators of the hip). Adaptation is our superpower—even if it's sometimes to a fault.

Core control isn't discussed extensively in this book, but it will be the next step in maximizing the activity you want to participate in, whether it be surfing for the first time or getting back into your pickup softball league. As a general principle, core work will bridge the gap from mobility to strength training.

Capacity—Strength-Training Principles 101

First, there are ways to combat the natural tendency to lose muscle and bone over time. One good way to accomplish this is through resistance training. The discussion in chapter 9 of age-related strength drop-off doesn't account for the positive effects of regularly putting your muscles through their paces. What you add in the gym can offset what nature subtracts. Being mobile in the absence of developing and maintaining muscle mass and strong bones isn't enough. If you've never lifted, start; and if you already have, keep going. Lifting doesn't necessarily mean hoisting a heavy barbell, either. You can also train your muscles with machines, hand weights, your own body weight (e.g., yoga, push-ups, step-ups, hiking), or resistance bands (e.g., Pilates reformer machines), forms of exercise already on the rise in popularity before the coronavirus pandemic made them home-workout essentials.

My philosophy is that everybody is different, and there is no one-size-fits-all routine. You must find the weight and reps that work for you based on who you are and what you're trying to accomplish. Switch things up, too. If you do the same routine every day, your body will grow used to it and you won't get any stronger. Your body is a lot smarter than you think, so you've got to force it to adapt to new demands. This is where capacity plays a role in training (one of my 3 C's in chapter 5). Capacity is the ability to handle increasing load demand. For example, take the classic push-up. You may possess the range of movement at the shoulders to complete the movement and the strength to do a full one. But how *many* can you do? Also, could you do them in slow motion (as occurs in yoga)? Can you do a clap push-up? The list goes on. The point is, capacity challenges the extent to which you can do a particular movement. It's the threshold required to progress your strength into different realms of movement.

Multi-joint and Multiplanar Movements

To make resistance training as helpful as possible in building muscle and bone strength, you should practice multi-joint movements in different planes, even though that approach is typically more challenging than simply performing isolation or single-joint movements. Take, for example, the traditional deadlift. This movement typically involves a proper lifting technique that utilizes the strength of your back, hips, knees, and feet. That's a *lot* of joints moving. But what about the *plane* of movement? The deadlift movement occurs on the sagittal plane (e.g., forward and backward), with minimal rotation. Traditionalists say to stay in this plane to minimize sheer. But how does this relate to functionality? Though a deadlift is challenging for the body, we rarely lift things in isolation in one plane of movement. Say you're trying to pick up your kid. Sometimes they are directly in front of you, but sometimes they're on your right or your left and you need to twist. Life is multiplanar with multiple joints. This practical and functional mind-set can lead to an unlimited amount of variation in your workouts.

An aspect of training smarter is recognizing and adapting to any vulnerable areas that have developed over the years. While you may have trained through aches and pains during your twenties or thirties and beyond, that mental and sometimes literal scar tissue racks up and should not be ignored. But what I *don't* want you to do is shy away from load. Load progression, as tolerated, is key. If your pain has improved and you want to go back to yoga, ease back into the movements you used to do. If it's not too painful getting into a plank, great! If it hurts after twenty seconds, then do two sets of ten-second planks. You can manipulate the load to work for you.

DO THIS NOW: Be mindful any time you lift something. Mindfulness has become a buzzword, and it's essential for maintaining long-term health and avoiding injuries. Don't be mindless when you ask your body to lift stuff. I can't tell you how many patients at Myodetox come to us after casually trying to lift a sofa or reaching down to grab something at an awkward angle, only to, boom, suffer an injury.

Think about what you're doing. In the sofa's case, square up with it, bend your knees, brace your core, and lift very deliberately. Better still, if you're middle-aged or older, do you really need to be lifting sofas or other heavy objects? It may lighten your wallet to hire someone, but your back will thank you.

Rest—Load Management and Care for Your Body

When will you know if you've trained too much or haven't rested enough? Simply put, pain is the best measure. Additionally, if you see a compromise in your quality of movement (like reduced mobility), then your body is hinting that it needs a break.

Regardless of how you train, don't hesitate to take a week off when you need it. That sort of break allows your body's systems to recover, including the central nervous system, skeletal muscles, tendons, and joints. When people get into training, they often feel like they can't miss a day without backsliding. But it takes a prolonged period of sloth for gains to just evaporate. *Never* taking off a few days—or even a week—can do more harm than good, especially if you have been training nonstop. When pounded daily, the body starts to wear down, and it gets harder and harder to recover. Remember, the body doesn't grow while a person lifts weights or sprints or cycles up a hill; it grows during the downtime. And too often, people minimize the latter.

As for when it's time to take a break, I hesitate to offer an exact cadence because everybody's different and everyone trains differently. One person might be training two or three times a week for thirty minutes a session, and they'll be in a much different state than somebody training seven days a week or getting ready for a marathon or obstacle race. There is no "one size fits all" when it comes to training or recovery. Listen closely to your body. Many people refer to instinctive training, but I also think *recovery* should be instinctive, too. If you find yourself worn down, irritable, or grumpy—or if you wake up tired—overtraining might be the culprit.

I mentioned earlier that pain and a breakdown of your form can indicate a need for rest. Typically, when you're seeing a decrease in your quality of movement (e.g., losing your balance, not being able to reach ranges of motion you typically hit, or experiencing discomfort and soreness earlier in an exercise), it's time to rest. You'll sacrifice your mobility and strength if you continually train without sufficient rest. For those who like more concrete guideposts, you may need to take a break if you find yourself breathless, feel chest pain, or experience a heightened heart rate even after rest.

Of course, there's much less of a need to take breaks from the posture and mobility regimen I've outlined here. When you're doing the Big Twelve, you're not hitting your muscles hard like you would during a weight workout or a hard grind on a cardio machine. Sure, you're moving your body through various ranges of motion, but at a low intensity. And because of that, you probably don't need to take a break—unless you need one because of mental fatigue or burnout. If the latter, don't let the Big Twelve vacation last too long. You've worked hard turning this routine into a habit, but habits can be broken.

Sleep: The Most Underrated Factor

When I was in physical therapy school, I would attend classes Monday through Friday and promote parties and events Thursday through Sunday. It was a crazy and unsustainable lifestyle. I'd host a lot of people, and I'd have to party with them. I'd go from table to table to see how everyone was doing, and they'd want me to take shots with them—which I'd fake. I'd say, "Hey, listen, I'll be right back," and I'd go find a room out of sight of everybody and study for half an hour. When I returned, I'd enthuse, "Isn't this party great?" And I'd fake-drink more shots before heading back for more study.

Somehow I managed to earn excellent grades, but in this lifestyle, sleep was the odd man out. I won an "award" for being the guy who slept most in class. Eventually, the lack of sleep catches up to you; it certainly caught up with me. I'm speaking from experience when I say that you can't futureproof your body without adequate sleep—seven or eight hours a night for most people. Sleep is when your muscles repair themselves, and it's when many vital hormones, including the male sex hormones, are released. It's also when the discs in your spine rehydrate and decompress.

Anabolic hormones—such as human growth factor—are unleashed in a cascade overnight. If you sleep only two or three hours, your muscles miss out on those growth factors. If you're deprived of sleep for any length of time, your body's ability to process glucose and hence produce energy is also short-circuited. Help yourself get quality sleep by winding down each day around the same time; also consider taking a hot bath, drinking herbal tea (avoid caffeine, though), and meditating.

Be Careful How You Sleep

Sleeping in the wrong position can undo the benefits of the Big Twelve. Many people go to bed feeling okay but wake up with a stiff, achy back; those with existing back pain often find it is worse upon waking. Things happen during sleep that affect spine health. Incorrect sleep posture might be the root cause of various spine issues.

There are three basic types of sleep posture:

▷ Side-lying

▷ Supine (facing up)

▷ Prone (facing down)

Is there one position that's ideal for everyone? It's impossible to generalize which sleep positions are better or worse for spine health and waking posture. Prone sleeping appears to place the most stress on the spine. Side sleeping tends to produce the fewest spine symptoms. Supine (on your back) sleeping is more of a mixed bag—okay for cervical but not so good for lumbar. Typically, a support is needed under the legs if you're going to sleep on your back. Side sleeping also tends to benefit those with obstructive sleep apnea, a breathing disorder with symptoms ranging from snoring to stoppages in breathing.

Bear in mind, most people change positions frequently throughout the night. Even healthy individuals change their sleep position ten to thirty times from the moment the lights get turned off to the instant the alarm buzzes. It might make sense to experiment with how you sprawl out as you tuck yourself in. If lying on your side, for example, seems to get you to sleep the fastest, that's something to try for a while. Of course, if you wake in the morning feeling horrible, that's an incentive to change things up the next time you're at the sleep start line.

If you feel your positioning is fine, but you're just not getting *enough* sleep, avoid late-night TV. A survey by the National Sleep Foundation found that half of adults borrow from sleep to watch television. Start dimming your lights the closer you get to bedtime. And try going to bed and waking at the same time every day, including weekends. A schedule helps reinforce the body's sleep-wake cycle, promoting better slumber.

11 TURNING PERFECT POSTURE INTO AN UNBREAKABLE HABIT

MOST PEOPLE FOLLOW routines for hygiene that were drummed into them as kids. They were told to take a bath or shower every day, shampoo their hair, brush their teeth after every meal, and change their underwear. At least initially, most parents don't even explain the health issues that arise from a lack of proper hygiene, whether it be cavities, dandruff, or a urinary tract infection. It's just what people *do*, they say. And when someone *doesn't* do it, they become the object of ridicule. No one at any age wants to become a social pariah because of poor hygiene.

As time passes, people's hygiene routines become more elaborate. They don't just shampoo; they add conditioner. Before brushing their teeth, they floss; afterward, they gargle. They moisturize after washing their face, trim their nails, maybe remove unwanted body hair.

When it comes to the spine and muscles, however, for most people it's out of sight, out of mind. Hopefully, if you've made it this far into the book, you're *not* going to be one of those people. I've given you a plan for promoting the hygiene of the spine and muscles—shown you how to futureproof your body. Now I want to make sure you turn that plan into an unbreakable habit.

There's a rule of thumb that it takes twenty-one days to create a new habit. That number has become a mantra in the fitness industry, where those who are out of shape try swapping their bad habits for good ones. Maybe they take up exercise because they see others being physically active and they want the same thing for themselves. So they set a goal of their own and embark on what they hope will be a successful transformation journey.

Unfortunately, the number of people who successfully transform themselves is a small fraction of those who begin. Large fitness websites can track the workout habits of those individuals who embark on a transformation, and it's crazy how many people, like clockwork, fall off the wagon during the third week. Apparently, people are embarrassed to quit after only a week, but at two weeks another factor may be kicking in. There may be an unrealistic need to *see* change taking place. "Surely something must be happening by *now*," a person tells him- or herself. People don't realize that while their *insides* may have changed for the better, it takes a bit longer for the *outside* to show all the work.

DO THIS NOW: Integrate this hygiene plan into your routine by starting small and building. What helps turn a goal-based behavior into a habit is making sure the action is fun, simple, efficient, and most of all, compatible with the rest of your life. Earlier in my career, I was one of those physical therapists who would give patients a notebook filled with twenty exercises to do at home as part of an hour-long regimen. It didn't work. They wouldn't do it.

In my experience, the best way for patients to develop healthy habits is to be taught slowly, with small wins building to bigger wins and significant progress. I don't give patients more than two exercises a week as homework. I'll say, "Work on those two things. I want you to do this every morning for me. Set a timer for five minutes, press go, and do it. That's it. Come back to see me and let me know how it went." Once they've integrated those two exercises into their routine, I'll give them two more—or a variation and upgrade of what they just did.

Not only do they tend to stick with this approach, but they start learning how their body works. By the end of our sessions, patients know how to manage their symptoms and pain.

This performance of habits is sometimes called automatic behavior, which is the opposite of reflective behavior. The more an action is repeated in response to a cue, the more habitual it becomes. As the name suggests, automatic behavior is much harder to inhibit, which can give it tremendous sway over someone's life. In the words of Will Durant, "We are what we repeatedly do." Habits help define us.

Let's be honest: Leaving your comfort zone and trying to change your behavior sucks, especially at the beginning. It's not fun. It's mentally draining. But it gets easier over time as the new habits take hold. Initially, you're going to have to use heaps of self-control and remind yourself and monitor your behavior, but eventually, performing the new action will become second nature. It won't take up as much mental capacity as when you started.

The great advantage of a habit is that by developing it, you have a better chance of sustaining long-term behavior change than if you simply rely on self-control. And by making automaticity your default, when your motivation wanes or you face a stressful situation or your priorities change, you won't give up and revert to your old habits.

The Habit of Sitting Too Much

Goal-directed behaviors and habits both rely on different neural networks and signaling processes within the brain. To demonstrate how intricate and delicate these systems are, think about people with obsessive-compulsive disorder, a dysfunction in the brain's habit network leading to overly rigid behaviors. It's not enough to wipe a doorknob before they touch it; they must wipe it twenty times every time.

DO THIS NOW: No matter what you do, keep up with your mobility training. It needs to be continuous, like brushing your teeth every day. It's not like you do it for a year and then call it good. This can be a challenge because slipping back into old habits is so easy. When you go out and accomplish great things, and you're busy and juggling multiple projects, sometimes it's tempting to let slip the very thing that has enabled you to do that. Don't take your eye off the ball. Don't take it for granted. Maintain your posture and mobility like a garden. You can water those plants for three or four years, and they'll look great. Stop for a year, and all that vegetation will die.

Once habits become established in the human brain circuitry, they're hard as hell to break—that is, unless the context for the cue changes. Let's say you've developed the habit of flossing your teeth daily, and the cue triggering the act is brushing your teeth before leaving the house each morning. After brushing comes flossing without a second thought.

DO THIS NOW: If you need some sort of reward initially to help form the habit of doing my routine, make it *simultaneous* with the routine rather than the cue to acting. A cup of coffee can be an effective cue, but if you must have that java as a reward to do the training, it probably won't last. Ideally, you want to get to where you're practicing the behavior because you value it and find it enjoyable. A better reward might be listening to your favorite music while you are performing the routine.

This can backfire, though. For example, when you relocate, the context for your cues changes. This probably won't disrupt your brushing and flossing habit because it's so basic and essential. The change in locations shouldn't be that big a deal. But the more complex the behavior, the more vulnerable it is when the context changes. Say you *do* move to a new home; your habitual exercise routine could be at risk. Going to the gym requires preparation: You have to put on the right clothes, and perhaps you need to fill your water bottle with a health drink. Then you have to get in the car and drive somewhere. Multicomponent behaviors like those are the hardest to turn into habits.

So how does sitting for many hours a day fit into this discussion? Well, think about it. Every morning, when you approach your desk or climb into your vehicle to begin a long day as a trucker, you don't weigh the pros and cons of sitting down. You just do it automatically. No, the habit you need to *instill* is taking multiple breaks from sitting down, which shouldn't be that difficult because regularly calling for a time-out doesn't involve multiple components.

Performing my posture hygiene routine every day is trickier. It's not like setting the timer on your watch to thirty minutes and getting up from your chair when the alarm buzzes and moving around and maybe doing some deep knee bends. My posture hygiene involves twelve discrete movements—even more if you want to add some of the variations. So how do you install that routine as a habit?

DO THIS NOW: Identify logical breaks between your tasks to get up and move. For example, tell yourself that you'll stand up and walk around a bit when you finish reviewing your email before doing anything else. Get a cup of coffee if you feel awkward randomly walking around the office. An unintended benefit of getting a beverage during your break is that it will make you pee, which will make you get up from your desk and walk again.

Just a minute ago, I mentioned that a possible way to avoid long bouts of sitting would be to set a timer on your phone so that an alarm goes off every thirty minutes reminding you to move around. The practice sounds foolproof, but humans have a way of resisting Pavlovian conditioning and simply choosing what they want to do

Katarzyna Stawarz, PhD, is a lecturer at Cardiff University in Wales specializing in human-computer interaction, a mixture of computer science and psychology. She has spent a lot of time studying apps to promote compliance for activities such as taking medications. This field of study interests me because I like the idea of your computer, smartphone, or other device reminding you to stand up and move around every thirty minutes or so. I also like the idea of similar prompts telling you to check your posture and sit up straight. "It's tricky because people learn to ignore the notifications," Stawarz told me. "What's more, if an alarm goes off every thirty minutes, it may come when you're in the middle of something, in which case you'll probably ignore it. It's easy to interrupt people and disrupt them. After a while, again, you'll learn to ignore it. This happens all the time in the studies we've done."

Stawarz and her associates have developed a prototype of a smarter app for reinforcing the habit of taking medications. The app's goal was to find specific things a user would do every day and employ them as triggers. For example, *Every time you eat your breakfast, take your pill.* Or *When you eat dinner, take your vitamin D supplement.* She suggests that similar techniques could be applied to an app for sitting less and moving more: *Whenever you finish a task, go for a walk.* An app is likelier to be more effective when it makes associations between elements of your routine. *Please remember to stretch after you get out of bed* is likely to be a more effective prompt than *Please remember to stretch.*

12 THE TIME TO START IS NOW

WHEN I WAS in my early twenties and in physical therapy school, I woke up one morning and felt a lump the size of a marble in the left side of my neck. It should have concerned me right then and there, but it didn't. When you're young, you think you're indestructible; you assume things like that will go away on their own—only this didn't. Instead, the marble grew to the size of a golf ball over a few months. Finally, I went to see a doctor, who sent me to an ear, nose, and throat specialist.

As it turned out, a tumor was growing in my throat. But it wasn't as simple as just cutting it out. First, it was dangerously close to my vocal cords. Second, it took numerous tests to determine if it was malignant, including having a needle the length of an iPhone Max stuck in my neck. Still, the results were inconclusive.

You can imagine how this all played with my mind. I was constantly anxious, always running my hand over the mass. One minute my brain would tell me it felt smaller; the next, that it felt bigger. It turns out the tumor inside my neck was growing and now blocked two-thirds of my carotid artery, the superhighway for blood entering the brain.

Finally, a surgeon gave me the bottom line: "Here's the deal," he said. "The tumor sits on your vagus nerve, which affects your heart, your lungs, and your left vocal cord. Your right vagus nerve would be able to take over heart duties from your left vagus, but your lungs will be affected and your left vocal cord will be paralyzed.

That said, if I don't take it out, you will most likely have a stroke. And while the mass isn't cancerous right now, as far we can tell, chances are it will be."

I remember walking outside on the street and bursting into tears. It was horrible to think I'd have speech problems at such a young age and run the risk of choking every time I drank water.

Fortunately, the surgery was successful. I was left with only a few minor residual issues: my left eyelid is droopy, my left pupil is smaller than the right, and I no longer sweat from the left side of my head. At the end of a hard workout, one side of my face is drenched while the other side is bone dry.

This close encounter with death at such a young age really shaped my mentality early on and shook me to the core. As hard as that experience was, it was mentally freeing in the end. It helped me see the fragility of life and understand the deep meaning of the cliché "Life is short." I no longer cared about what others thought about me from that moment on, which helped me think outside the box when creating Myodetox. I became acutely aware that "health is wealth," that nothing else mattered when you were sick.

The reason I wrote this book is so that other people will have those same realizations: that life is short and that the choices you make early on, whether it's poor posture or poor movement habits, have consequences down the road. Even though this book is titled *Sit Up Straight*, its point is not to tell you to sit up straight 24/7. When I ask you to sit up straight, what I'm really asking you to do is PAY ATTENTION—not only to how you sit, but to how you move, how you speak, how you live your life. So many people are on autopilot and watch time fly by instead of truly living. They let life lead them instead of leading their life.

Learning about your body, how it works and how it moves, is a lifelong journey. Don't let that reality frustrate you; that's what makes it all so rewarding in the end.

If you follow my plan consistently, the compounding effects are profound. Following a program like this is about removing roadblocks from your path. I'm talking about barriers like injuries, chronic pain, and disability. Although accidents may happen and life stressors may lead to pain or tension in your body, remember that your body is resilient. By following this program you'll be back on track to a healthy and pain-free life.

You've taken the first important step by merely reading this book. Now it's time to take what you've learned and put it into action every day, every week, every month, every year.

SOURCES

MUCH OF THE INFORMATION in this book comes from my professional studies over the years, the coursework people like me undertake to become certified and begin practicing physical therapy. Beyond that, my theories are based on an in-depth and ongoing review of the scientific literature. Science changes all the time; someone who earns a certificate and doesn't look at a new study for several years is already hopelessly behind. My views are also informed, inevitably, by my personal experiences with thousands of clients seen during fourteen years of practice. This empirical research is essential and invaluable, as long as it's viewed and validated through the prism of the aforementioned research.

1. Posture, Pain, and a Pandemic

5   "Individuals with chronic pain": M. Racine. "Chronic Pain and Suicide Risk: A Comprehensive Review." *Progress in Neuro-Psychopharmacology & Biological Psychiatry* 87, pt. B (2018): 269–80. doi: 10.1016/j.pnpbp.2017.08.020.

5   a billion-dollar industry, with 70 percent of U.S. adults: D. Rubin. "Epidemiology and Risk Factors for Spine Pain." *Neurologic Clinics* 25, no. 2 (2007): 353–71. doi: 10.1016/j .ncl.2007.01.004.

12   one in six people worldwide will be over age sixty-five: United Nations, Department of Economic and Social Affairs, Population Division. *World Population Prospects 2019: Highlights* (ST/ESA/SER.A/423).

2. The Blueprint of Your Body's Posture

24   the energy expended by those who are sitting compared to: S. A. Creasy et al. "Energy Expenditure During Acute Periods of Sitting, Standing, and Walking." *Journal of Physical Activity and Health* 13, no. 6 (2016): 573–78. doi: 10.1123/jpah.2015-0419.

25   getting up and standing for at least *half* the time you're at work: Brigid Schulte. "Economic Policy: Health Experts Have Figured Out How Much You Should Sit Each Day." *Washington Post,* June 2, 2015. https://www.washingtonpost.com/news/wonk/wp/2015/06/02 /medical-researchers-have-figured-out-how-much-time-is-okay-to-spend-sitting-each-day/.

40   the costs of a sedentary lifestyle: D. Ding et al. "The Economic Burden of Physical Inactivity: A Global Analysis of Major Non-Communicable Diseases." *The Lancet* 388, no. 10051 (2016): 1311–24. doi: 10.1016/S0140-6736(16)30383-X.

41   one in four Americans sits for more than eight hours a day: E. N. Ussery et al. "Joint Prevalence of Sitting Time and Leisure-Time Physical Activity Among US Adults, 2015– 2016." *JAMA* 320, no. 19 (2018): 2036–38.

41   study comparing transit drivers: J. N. Morris et al. "Coronary Heart-Disease and Physical Activity of Work." *The Lancet* 262, no. 6795 (1953): 1053–57. doi: 10.1016/s0140 -6736(53)90665-5.

41   In a meta-analysis of more than 1 million people: U. Ekelund et al. "Does Physical Activity Attenuate, or even Eliminate, the Detrimental Association of Sitting Time with Mortality? A Harmonised Meta-Analysis of Data from More Than 1 Million Men and Women." *The Lancet* 388, no. 10051 (2016): 1302–10. doi: 10.1016/S0140-6736(16)30370-1.

41   6 percent of all deaths worldwide can be attributed to inactivity: "Global Health Risks: Mortality and Burden of Disease Attributable to Selected Major Risks." Geneva: World Health Organization, 2009.

42   On average teens use their smartphone: "The Common Sense Census: Media Use by Tweens and Teens, 2019." https://www.commonsensemedia.org/research/the-common -sense-census-media-use-by-tweens-and-teens-2019. This report presents the results of a nationally representative survey of more than 1,600 U.S. eight- to eighteen-year-olds, about their use of and relationship with media.

3. Sixteen Health Landmines Related to Bad Posture

48   Having more weight around your waist: N. Teasdale et al. "Obesity Alters Balance and Movement Control." *Current Obesity Reports* 2, no. 3 (2013): 235–40. doi:10.1007/s13679-013-0057-8.

48   The older someone gets, the more pronounced: J. Giannoudis, C. A. Bailey, and R. M. Daly. "Associations Between Sedentary Behaviour and Body Composition, Muscle

Function and Sarcopenia in Community-Dwelling Older Adults." *Osteoporosis International* 26, no. 2 (2015): 571–79. doi: 10.1007/s00198-014-2895-y.

49   physical activity reduces the rate of bone loss: R. Nikander et al. "Targeted Exercise Against Osteoporosis: A Systematic Review and Meta-Analysis for Optimising Bone Strength Throughout Life." *BMC Medicine* 8, no. 47 (2010). doi: 10.1186/1741-7015-8-47.

49   Hunched posture and too much sitting weakens postural muscles: E-Y. Kim, K-J. Kim, and H-R. Park. "Comparison of the Effects of Deep Neck Flexor Strengthening Exercises and Mackenzie Neck Exercises on Head Forward Postures Due to the Use of Smartphones." *Indian Journal of Science and Technology* 8, suppl. 7 (2015): 569–75. doi: 10.17485/ijst/2015 /v8iS7/70462.

55   An Iranian study found that staring at a computer: P. Nejati, S. Loftian, A. Moezy, and M. Nejati. "The Study of Correlation Between Forward Head Posture and Neck Pain in Iranian Office Workers." *International Journal of Occupational Medicine and Environmental Health* 28, no. 2 (2015): 295–303. doi: 10.13075/ijomeh.1896.00352.

56   neck pain ranged from 28 to 61 percent: N. Pargali and N. Jowkar. "Prevalence of Musculoskeletal Pain Among Dentists in Shiraz, Southern Iran." *International Journal of Occupational and Environmental Medicine* 1, no. 2 (2010): 69–74; A. Aarabi et al. "Musculoskeletal Disorders in Dentists in Shiraz, Southern Iran." *Iranian Red Crescent Medical Journal* 11, no. 4 (2009): 464–65; G. Chamani et al. "Prevalence of Musculoskeletal Disorders Among Dentists in Kerman, Iran." *Journal of Musculoskeletal Pain* 20, no. 3 (2012): 202–7. doi: 10.3109/10582452.2012.704138.

57   a rounded mid back can increase your risk for a tendon tear: A. Yamamoto et al. "The Impact of Faulty Posture on Rotator Cuff Tears with and without Symptoms." *Journal of Shoulder and Elbow Surgery* 24, no. 3 (2015): 446–52. doi: 10.1016/j.jse.2014.07.012.

58   tend to adopt a hunched posture: A. Cuddy. "Your iPhone Is Ruining Your Posture—and Your Mood." *New York Times* online, December 12, 2015. https://www.nytimes.com/2015 /12/13/opinion/sunday/your-iphone-is-ruining-your-posture-and-your-mood.html.

59   a more difficult time pulling themselves out of a bad mood: L. Veenstra, I. K. Schneider, and S. L. Koole. "Embodied Mood Regulation: The Impact of Body Posture on Mood Recovery, Negative Thoughts, and Mood-Congruent Recall." *Cognition and Emotion* 31, no. 7 (2017): 1361–76. doi: 10.1080/02699931.2016.1225003.

59   Eight out of ten U.S. adults say they experience stress: L. Saad. "8 in 10 Americans Afflicted by Stress." Gallup Wellbeing, December 20, 2017. Gallup poll based on telephone interviews conducted December 4–11, 2017, with a random sample of 1,049 adults, aged eighteen and older, living in all fifty U.S. states and the District of Columbia. https://news.gallup.com /poll/224336/eight-americans-afflicted-stress.aspx.

60   sedentary behavior elevates the risk of insomnia: Y. Yang et al. "Sedentary Behavior and Sleep Problems: A Systematic Review and Meta-Analysis." *International Journal of Behavioral Medicine* 24, no. 4 (2017): 481–92. doi: 10.1007/s12529-016-9609-0.

61   falls are the leading cause of injuries among the elderly: Centers for Disease Control and Prevention, "Keep on Your Feet—Preventing Older Adult Falls." https://www.cdc.gov /injury/features/older-adult-falls/index.html.

62   the elderly often lose their ability to move laterally: M. J. Hilliard et al. "Lateral Balance Factors Predict Future Falls in Community-Living Older Adults." *Archives of Physical Medicine and Rehabilitation* 89, no. 9 (2008): 1708–13. doi: 10.1016/j.apmr.2008.01.023.

62   A slouched or collapsed sitting posture compresses the lungs: Sarah Dalton; reviewed by Judith Marcin, MD. "Breathe Deeper to Improve Health and Posture." Healthline, August 18, 2020. https://www.healthline.com/health/breathe-deeper-improve-health-and-posture.

4. Movement Is Life

69   the "stitching" that holds together: C. Stecco et al. "The Fascia: The Forgotten Structure." *Italian Journal of Anatomy and Embryology* 116, no. 3 (2011): 127–38.

71   Applying intentional specific mechanical stress: N. R. Dhiman et al. "Myofascial Release Versus Other Soft Tissue Release Techniques Along Superficial Back Line Structures for Improving Flexibility in Asymptomatic Adults: A Systematic Review with Meta-Analysis." *Journal of Bodywork and Movement Therapies* 28 (2021): 450–57. doi: 10.1016/j.jbmt.2021.06.026.

75   static stretches can actually *decrease*: J. Opplert and N. Babault. "Acute Effects of Dynamic Stretching on Muscle Flexibility and Performance: An Analysis of the Current Literature." *Sports Medicine* 48, no. 2 (2018): 299–325. doi: 10.1007/s40279-017-0797-9.

5. Understanding Where You Stand

86   an injury can change proprioception: M. J. Rivera, Z. K. Winkelmann, C. J. Powden, and K. E. Games. "Proprioceptive Training for the Prevention of Ankle Sprains: An Evidence-Based Review." *Journal of Athletic Training* 52, no. 11 (2017): 1065–67. doi: 10.4085/1062-6050-52.11.16.

87   proprioceptive input at the trunk: J. E. Aman, N. Elangovan, I-L. Yeh, and J. Konczak. "The Effectiveness of Proprioceptive Training for Improving Motor Function: A Systematic Review." *Frontiers in Human Neuroscience* 8 (2014): 1075. doi: 10.3389/fnhum.2014.01075.

7. Foam Rolling for Next-Level Mobility

141   improve flexibility: S. W. Cheatham, M. J. Kolber, M. Cain, and M. Lee. "The Effects of Self-Myofascial Release Using a Foam Roll or Roller Massager on Joint Range of Motion,

Muscle Recovery, and Performance: A Systematic Review." *International Journal of Sports Physical Therapy* 10, no. 6 (2015): 827–38.

153   These slings comprise muscle: M. Panjabi. "The Stabilizing System of the Spine. Part I. Function, Dysfunction, Adaptation, and Enhancement." *Journal of Spinal Disorders* 5, no. 4 (1992): 383–89. doi: 10.1097/00002517-199212000-00001.

8. Ten Common Health Ailments Solved

160   Tension and cervicogenic headaches can be influenced: P. R. Blanpied et al. "Neck Pain: Revision 2017: Clinical Practice Guidelines Linked to the International Classification of Functioning, Disability, and Health from the Orthopaedic Section of the American Physical Therapy Association." *Journal of Orthopaedic & Sports Physical Therapy* 47, no. 7 (2017): A1–A83. doi: 10.2519/jospt.2017.0302.

161   This is why conditions like carpal tunnel syndrome: A. I. De-la-Llave-Rincón, C. Fernandez-de-las-Peñas, D. Palacios-Ceña, and J. A. Cleland. "Increased Forward Head Posture and Restricted Cervical Range of Motion in Patients with Carpal Tunnel Syndrome." *Journal of Orthopaedic & Sports Physical Therapy* 39, no. 9 (2009): 658–64. doi: 10.2519/jospt.20009.3058.

161   thoracic outlet syndrome can manifest from the neck: N. A. Levine and B. R. Rigby. "Thoracic Outlet Syndrome: Biomechanical and Exercise Considerations." *Healthcare* (Basel) 6, no. 2 (2018): 68. doi: 10.3390/healthcare6020068.

166   twice as prevalent in men than women: O. R. Fjeld et al. "Complications, Reoperations, Readmissions, and Length of Hospital Stay in 34,639 Surgical Cases of Lumbar Disc Herniation." *Bone & Joint Journal* 101-B, no. 4 (2019): 470–77. doi: 10.1302/0301-620X.101B4.BJJ-2018-1184.R1.

166   mobility and exercise have been shown to be effective in mitigating: W. Xu et al. "Is Lumbar Fusion Necessary for Chronic Low Back Pain Associated with Degenerative Disc Disease? A Meta-Analysis." *World Neurosurgery* 146 (2021): 298–306. doi: 10.1016/j.wneu.2020.11.121.

166   up to 30 percent of disc herniations: W. Brinjikji et al. "MRI Findings of Disc Degeneration Are More Prevalent in Adults with Low Back Pain Than in Asymptomatic Controls: A Systematic Review and Meta-Analysis." *American Journal of Neuroradiology* 36, no. 12 (2015): 2394–99. doi: 10.3174/ajnr.A4498.

170   It's an overuse injury related to repetitive stress: D. Sisk and M. Fredericson. "Update of Risk Factors, Diagnosis, and Management of Patellofemoral Pain." *Current Reviews in Musculoskeletal Medicine* 12, no. 3 (2019): 534–41. doi: 10.1007/s12178-019-09593-z.

170   two bosses: the hip: C. J. Barton, S. Lack, P. Malliaras, and D. Morrissey. "Gluteal Muscle Activity and Patellofemoral Pain Syndrome: A Systematic Review." *British Journal of Sports Medicine* 47, no. 4 (2013): 207–14. doi: 10.1136/bjsports-2012-090953.

170 and the foot: D. Sisk and M. Fredericson. "Update of Risk Factors, Diagnosis, and Management of Patellofemoral Pain." *Current Reviews in Musculoskeletal Medicine* 12, no. 4 (2019): 534–41. doi: 10.1007/s12178-019-09593-z.

171 poor foot mobility and walking mechanics: J. D. Goff and R. Crawford. "Diagnosis and Treatment of Plantar Fasciitis." *American Family Physician* 84, no. 6 (2011): 676–82; L. Luffy, J. Grosel, R. Thomas, and E. So. "Plantar Fasciitis: A Review of Treatments." *Journal of the American Academy of Physician Assistants* 31, no. 1 (2018), 20–24. doi: 10.1007 /s12178-019-09593-z.

174 80 percent of people in America: J. K. Freburger et al. "The Rising Prevalence of Chronic Low Back Pain." *Archives of Internal Medicine* 169, no. 3 (2009): 251–58. doi: 10.1001 /archinternmed.2008.543.

9. The Challenges Facing Specific Groups

178 Erik Dalton, PhD, a manual therapist, educator, and author: E. Dalton, "Puzzle of Perfect Posture." From Advanced Upper Body course. https://erikdalton.com/blog/puzzle -perfect-posture/.

178 NASA has extensively researched the changes: M. Stavnichuk et al. "A Systematic Review and Meta-Analysis of Bone Loss in Space Travelers." *Nature Partner Journals: Microgravity* 13 (2020).

179 it leads to greater curvature: C. Roux et al. "Prospective Assessment of Thoracic Kyphosis in Postmenopausal Women with Osteoporosis." *Journal of Bone and Mineral Research* 25, no. 2 (2010): 362–68. doi: 10.1359/jbmr.090727.

179 Medications like steroids: F. Pouresmaeili, B. Kamalidehghan, M. Kamarehei, and Y. M. Goh. "A Comprehensive Overview on Osteoporosis and Its Risk Factors." *Therapeutics and Clinical Risk Management* 14 (2018): 2029–49. doi: 10.2147/TCRM.S138000.

179 200 million people in the world: T. Sozen, L. Özisik, and N. C. Basaran. "An Overview and Management of Osteoporosis." *European Journal of Rheumatology* 4, no. 1 (2017): 46–56. doi: 10.5152/eurjrheum.2016.048.

179 as women age, the prevalence of osteoporosis increases: S. S-T. Lo. "Prevalence of Osteoporosis in Elderly Women in Hong Kong." *Osteoporosis and Sarcopenia* 7, no. 3 (2021): 92–97. doi: 10.1016/j.afos.2021.09.001.

180 falls account for nearly 300,000 hip fractures: Centers for Disease Control and Prevention. "Hip Fractures Among Older Adults, 2016." https://www.cdc.gov/homeandrecreationalsafety /falls/adulthipfx.html.

180 physical therapy intervention can reduce falls: S. Karinkanta et al. "Physical Therapy Approaches to Reduce Fall and Fracture Risk Among Older Adults." *Nature Review: Endocrinology* 6, no. 7 (2010): 396–407. doi: 10.1038/nrendo.2010.70.

180   starting around age thirty: T. G. Travison et al. "Harmonized Reference Ranges for Circulating Testosterone Levels in Men of Four Cohort Studies in the United States and Europe." *Journal of Clinical Endocrinology and Metabolism* 102, no. 4 (2017): 1161–73. doi: 10.1210/jc.2016-2935.

180   Along with the back muscles, the glutes: N. A. Cooper et al. "Prevalence of Gluteus Medius Weakness in People with Chronic Low Back Pain Compared to Health Controls." *European Spine Journal* 25, no. 4 (2016): 1258–65. doi:10.1007/s00586-015-4027-6.

181   Strength peaks at roughly twenty-five: E. Volpi, R. Nazemi, and S. Fujita. "Muscle Tissue Changes with Aging." *Current Opinion in Clinical Nutrition & Metabolic Care* 7, no. 4 (2004): 405–10. doi: 10.1097/01.mco.0000134362.76653.b2.

182   women are more prone than men to neck and shoulder symptoms: R. Fejer, K. O. Kyvik, and J. Hartvigsen. "The Prevalence of Neck Pain in the World Population: A Systematic Critical Review of the Literature." *European Spine Journal* 15, no. 6 (2005): 834–48. doi: 10.1007/s00586-004-0864-4.

182   issues related to using touchscreen devices: S. H. Toh, P. Coenen, E. K. Howie, and L. M. Straker. "The Associations of Mobile Touch Screen Device Use with Musculoskeletal Symptoms and Exposures: A Systematic Review." *PLoS ONE* 12, no. 8 (2017): e0181220. doi: 10.1371/journal.pone.0181220.

182   Women are even more likely than men to experience low back pain: A. Delitto et al. "Low Back Pain: Clinical Practice Guidelines Linked to the International Classification of Functioning, Disability, and Health from the Orthopaedic Section of the American Physical Therapy Association." *Journal of Orthopaedic & Sports Physical Therapy* 42, no. 4 (2012): A1–A57. https://www.jospt.org/doi/10.2519/jospt.2012.42.4.A1.

183   were literally peeing during heavy lifts: CrossFit, "Do You Pee During Workouts?" https://www.youtube.com/watch?v=UKzq1upNIgU.

183   up to 90 percent of women who experience low back pain: S. Dufour, B. Vandyken, M-J. Forget, and C. Vandyken. "Association Between Lumbopelvic Pain and Pelvic Floor Dysfunction in Women: A Cross Sectional Study." *Musculoskeletal Science and Practice* 34 (2018): 47–53. doi: 10.1016/l.msksp.2017.12.001.

183   I recommend that if you do experience any of the above symptoms: I. Nygaard et al. "Prevalence of Symptomatic Pelvic Floor Disorders in US Women." *Journal of the American Medical Association* 300, no. 11 (2008): 1311–16. doi: 10.1001/jama.300 .11.1311.

186   Women tend to have more significant lumbar lordosis: O. Hay et al. "The Lumbar Lordosis in Males and Females, Revisited." *PLoS One* 10, no. 8 (2015): e0133685. doi: 10.1371 /journal.pone.0133685.

186 those with "flat back": J. Beck, H. Brisby, A. Baranto, and O. Westin. "Low Lordosis Is a Common Finding in Young Lumbar Disc Herniation Patients." *Journal of Experimental Orthopaedics* 7 (2020): 38. doi: 10.1186/s40634-020-00253-7.

186 gluteus maximus and gluteus medius muscles: N. A. Cooper et al. "Prevalence of Gluteus Medius Weakness in People with Chronic Low Back Pain Compared to Healthy Controls." *European Spine Journal* 25, no. 4 (2016): 1258–65. doi:10.1007/s00586-015-4027-6.

187 But as I mentioned earlier, pelvic floor dysfunction: A. H. MacLennan, A. W. Taylor, D. H. Wilson, and D. Wilson. "The Prevalence of Pelvic Floor Disorders and Their Relationship to Gender, Age, Parity, and Mode of Delivery." *British Journal of Obstetrics and Gynaecology* 107, no. 12 (2000): 1460–70. doi: 10.1111/j.1471-0528.2000.tb11669.x.

187 nearly 80 percent will report an injury to a lower extremity: M. P. van der Worp et al. "Injuries in Runners: A Systematic Review on Risk Factors and Sex Differences." *PLoS One* 10, no. 2 (2015): e0114937. doi: 10.1371/journal.pone.0114937.

ACKNOWLEDGMENTS

Like building a brand, writing a book is a team effort from start to finish. I want to take a moment to thank some significant contributors.

Jeff O'Connell and Nathan Santos were instrumental in helping me write and research *Sit Up Straight*. Without their contributions, the information in the book would still be random ideas floating around in my brain. Thank you for helping me bring my vision to life.

Big thanks as well to Andrew Sabarre, Aaron Cooper, Yu-King Wong, Michael Bercasio, Sophia Chang, Judith Humphrey, and Robert Greene, for taking the time to read and critique the book as it came to life. The finished product benefited greatly from your criticisms and insights.

I also must give a major shoutout (and kisses) to Kayla Hamm for supporting me through this stressful process and giving me invaluable insights. Love you!

Thank you to my agents Marc Gerald and Tess Callero of Europa Content for "discovering" me on the Nike podcast and believing in me from the jump. You were indispensable guides on my first book.

To my illustrator, Josh Klein, thank you for being patient with us as the project evolved. I'm grateful and blessed to have your talent forever imprinted in this book.

To Julian Nieva, thank you for acing the book's photography. Your experience and hard work made a huge difference. The photoshoots were so smooth and well organized. And I can't lie, you made something that could have been mundane so much fun.

To Anil Mohambir and Mike Orquia, thank you so much for being so gracious with your studios. Having access to your beautiful spaces made the process and the results that much better.

To the models, thank you for lending your good looks (it was an honor to witness your Blue Steels) and good energy to the set.

Othello Grey, Nam Phi Dang, Ja Tecson—thank you for contributing your photography skills to this project.

To Rick Horgan, Olivia Bernhard, and the whole crew at Simon & Schuster— thank you for believing in me, green-lighting this project, and helping me bring it to life!

To Mom and Dad, if it weren't for you raising me to be a good man and instilling in me a strong work ethic, I wouldn't be where I am today. I hope this book makes you proud.

To everyone else who contributed to the book, I sincerely thank you.

And finally, to all my past patients and the Myodetox community, I want to thank you for inspiring me to write this book. I hope you all enjoy it because it was inspired by you and created for you. Love you all!